My Reluctant Journey

Lessons Learned on the Path to Retirement

Dr. Edy Stoughton PhD

Copyright © 2015 Dr. Edy Stoughton PhD
All rights reserved.

ISBN: 1511903139
ISBN 13: 9781511903134

Acknowledgements

I COULD NEVER have written this book without the support of some very special people. One of the most important lessons I learned through this process is that this is a journey we must take together. My husband, Steve, has been my partner in every endeavor I have undertaken throughout our 48 years of married life. His patience and wisdom keep me going and make the journey special and joyful. My children Jason, Craig, Chris, Amanda and Abigail along with their amazing partners Julie, Carolina, Mike and Beau are the most insightful and supportive people I have ever known. Their feedback and belief in me are both invaluable and deeply appreciated. To my grandchildren, Ana, Nate, Campbell, Lauren and Elle—you are the reason I do what I do. You are smart and funny and you fill me with joy. Finally, this book would never have been written without my group of wonderful friends who believe in the truth and relevance to their experience of this project. They read and reread drafts, offered wise suggestions and never let me quit. To Vicki, Barb, Sharon, Sally, Terri and Sue Anne, my partners on this journey, I am so grateful for your support and guidance.

Table of Contents

Acknowledgements		iii
Foreward		vii
Chapter 1	Stepping Out Into Thin Air	1
Chapter 2	Every Journey Starts With a Single Step-- But In What Direction?	13
Chapter 3	Who Am I Really?	16
Chapter 4	The Best-Laid Plans	20
Chapter 5	Taking Stock	30
Chapter 6	Revisiting That Spiritual/Human Connection	39
Chapter 7	Forward Momentum in a Positive Direction	42
Chapter 8	Is There a Pattern Here?	46

Chapter 9 "Guts and Honor"	52
Chapter 10 Walking Through New Doors	57
Chapter 11 Claiming my Inner Strength	67
Chapter 12 Roots and Wings: Cherish the Past but Keep Growing	77
Chapter 13 The Only Good Place to Live is Outside the Box	82
Chapter 14 A Year of Challenges, Growth, and Joy	91
About the Author	109

Foreword

ON MAY 20, 2015 David Letterman exited the stage from a career as an entertainment icon that has spanned over 30 years. Right before this momentous date he was interviewed by Jane Pauley. During the course of that interview he said that he felt "naked and afraid" about retiring from the Tonight show. To many people that was a surprising response. Certainly his position and the financial security that accompanies it will allow him to do pretty much whatever he wants. But what he was feeling when he spoke candidly during that interview goes beyond that. My guess is that what he is facing is that he is no longer who he has been and now he must begin the hard work of deciding who he will become. He expressed during that same interview his concern about what lies ahead when he said that after leaving the show he had hosted for so many years, "I don't think anyone will ever see me again."

This is the same worry expressed by a friend of mine who is also on the edge of retirement. One evening we met for dinner and I asked him how he was doing. He shot back, "I feel invisible." Although he is not a celebrity, my friend is struggling with the same psychic questions of "Who am I now?" "Where am I heading?" and "Will my life still have meaning?"

This book is a chronicle of my search for answers to these questions. My journey is becoming more common as women are retiring in increasing numbers from careers that have provided an important sense of meaning and identity. One of the biggest minefields lies in not knowing what to expect. That is why I wrote this book for women. There are not an abundance of examples of how previous generations of women handled retirement because many of them didn't have professional lives and so didn't retire. We will be the examples for women who follow us in transitioning from a career to a post-career life. It is my hope that this book will add to the conversation we must have about how we will find joy and fulfillment and purpose in retirement as we traverse this often reluctant journey.

1

Stepping Out Into Thin Air
**1 Month Into My Life of Retirement
August, 2013**

*"When I let go of what I am, I become
what I might be."*

— Lao Tze

"RETIREMENT ISN'T AN event, it's a process." I have heard these words of wisdom many times and I believe they are true. Yet, at this point, the process isn't going very smoothly for me. One month ago I retired. I smiled through my retirement party, said my goodbyes and packed the car to drive with my husband and dog to our vacation home in Michigan with the plan being to thoughtfully contemplate our next steps before launching our new life. Doing nothing was definitely not one of the options I would be contemplating. I empathize with the words of Jennifer Granholm who, when asked what she was going to do upon leaving the governorship of Michigan replied, "Sit on a beach and drink Margaritas." After a lifetime of working hard, a little beach time sounds appealing. But that lifestyle would wear thin fairly quickly for me as I expect it would for Ms. Granholm. But doing nothing seems to be exactly what I am doing right now. I believed that when I retired I would take a short breather to regroup and then

I would choose from among a number of interesting options to find something fun and engaging to do. I was unprepared for the emotional adjustment when my phone stopped ringing, my inbox wasn't full, and no opportunities were knocking on my door.

When I need to figure things out, I write about them. So I am beginning this journal to attempt to make sense out of what I am experiencing, untangle my confusing emotions and figure out a way forward. In addition, to be completely honest, I need to have something to do. This journey is just beginning for me and it is such new and unfamiliar terrain that I don't even know how I want it to go. But I have learned that sometimes the most interesting situation to be in is this area of perplexity. With Lao Tze's words to guide me, I hope to keep my mind open to face whatever is in store with my mind open to the possibilities, whatever they may be. And so the journey begins.

Most of us engage in some sort of "retirement prep" in which we rehearse what our life will be when we are no longer a regular part of the working world. Very rarely does it come as a surprise to any of us in our 60s that we are rapidly reaching the point when it is time to move out of the stressful, demanding working life that we have inhabited for so many years. If we chance to forget, our bosses, boards of directors, and particularly those younger co-workers who aspire to move up into our positions will make sure we don't ignore this reality for long. And this is as it should be. I feel that there is a certain lack of awareness and "tone deafness" in hanging on in a position too long when it has become clear that it is time for a change. Giving those who are coming behind us a chance to shine can be the right thing to do. That "right time" certainly shouldn't be solely based on chronological age, but it is one of the considerations.

To reach the new aging demographic (us), the media is increasingly featuring ads that show attractive and obviously happy older people enjoying the rewarding, active-yet-relaxed post-work life that we are assured we too can have. We begin dreaming about our own next step. But all of this tends to remain at a hazy level of "someday" as most of us procrastinate when it comes to thinking very deeply and honestly about the future and our own inevitable aging. I clearly remember both my husband and me repeating breezily through the years, "We're never going to retire" with our thought being (when we even gave it any thought) that when the right time came we would naturally transition into the "perfect" job where we would still be in the midst of things but on our own terms. I think we still subconsciously cling to that idea. That sort of evolution can happen. Some people I know have made a largely seamless transition from a full-time profession to a less demanding version of that job oftentimes within the same organization. They just go from being the "sage on the stage" to the "wise elder statesman." However, those people generally started pretty early on planning purposefully much like those who begin saving on their 401k plans at the onset of their working lives rather than scrambling to start saving when the shadows are lengthening.

Throughout my life I have sought out, and thrived on, challenges. My drive to prove myself has been relentless and my biggest fear has been that there would not be enough time to accomplish all that I wanted to do. One time I participated in a conversation-starter at a professional event in which we were asked to answer the familiar question, "If you knew this was the last day of your life, what would be your biggest regret?" I had no trouble answering the question. My biggest regret without a doubt would be to think of the things I wish I had done but had put off until it was too late.

At 22 years old with my brand new sociology degree in hand, I accepted a social work job in the section of my city (Indianapolis) that topped the charts for violent crime. A few years later, I taught students labeled "emotionally disturbed" and considered too troubled to be in the general school population in a self-contained classroom. I enrolled in Indiana University to get my doctorate when I was 52 years old. Upon earning my doctorate I accepted a one-year visiting appointment at Teacher's College, Columbia University living in a Manhattan apartment by myself and experiencing the city. My husband visited on weekends and it was a great adventure. Recently I was Head of School for Midwest Academy, a private school specializing in students with Asperger's syndrome. During my leadership, I brought the school from the brink of financial ruin to success and accreditation. Although these past experiences were challenging as well as demanding, I can safely say that at this point in my life I am facing the toughest challenge yet—retirement.

In retrospect, I don't think I was fully ready for it. Is anyone ever really ready for this time of life? But I knew it was time. For 7 years I had run the school. I loved my job and felt privileged to be able to do such fulfilling and rewarding work with people I truly cared about. It was wonderful seeing the difference in the lives of the students and I was proud of the special school I had built. I didn't feel I would be departing with unfinished business. The school was in good shape and I knew I was leaving a thriving legacy behind. But, sadly, my late-60s body had begun to send me unmistakable messages. I was becoming physically, mentally and emotionally drained, feeling less eager to rush into work to face the day and more reluctant to stay into the evening. In short, I was tired. This was in addition to the fact that we would be moving into a new building to accommodate our growing enrollment. All the fund raising and tense, hard work the move would entail made this seem to be a good time to make a transition in my own life. In addition, I was feeling badly that I seemed to always be working when my family wanted to spend time with me. Finally, I longed to spend more time with my husband in the vacation home that we loved located on Lake Michigan. So I entered a period of psychic conflict. I had a heady life running a school. My opinions were listened to and acted upon. I was able to make decisions that had positive effects on families' lives. In my own sphere I was "important" and I was making a difference. I loved what I did. And yet it was clear that it would have to end sometime. Nothing ever stays static, change is inevitable. The question seemed to be, **"Was that time now and was I ready for it?"** I wrote in my journal, lay awake making mental lists of pros and cons and had deep, heartfelt conversations with my family and friends. One of my journal entries read, for example: "I don't seem to have as much passion and fire anymore. Passion and fire were always my hallmarks. I have always been driven and full of energy and now I'm really not." There were many "pros." High on the list were spending more time in our Michigan home which had always been a special retreat and where I believe I am my most authentic self; being an involved part of my grandchildren's lives as they grow up; delving into some projects and activities that I had put on the back burner; and taking better care of my health and well-being. But there were some definite "cons", most important of which was the question of what it really means to be retired. I would be stepping out into unfamiliar territory with no chance for a "do over." There was no way that once the decision had been made I would be able to go back and say I had changed my mind. To a great extent my career had defined me. Would I lose my identity, disappearing into a world of meaningless and sedentary pursuits? Would I become invisible? Basically, would I become "old?"

Another issue to wrestle with was one that also seemed like a positive thing, but that I was now finding to be a mixed blessing. What I am referring to is the new catch phrase that "60 is the new 50." We've all heard this and at first blush it sounds really cool. How lucky we are to be living in a time when we are able to cheat the natural aging process without even lifting a finger. But the whole idea is somewhat of a slippery slope. At one time, not too long ago, there were pretty clear rules about how the passages of our lives should go. There was a mandatory retirement age, or at least a common understanding, and no one believed that when they were 80 they were really 70. Of course there was a certain harshness and inevitability about the commonly accepted "ages and stages", but at least you knew what you were dealing with. The problem with the new thinking is that we can feel inadequate if we really do feel and look 60 rather than 40. So we worry and work very hard at being young. Another thing is that without mandatory retirement we worry about whether it is the "right" time or not. At least that was certainly true for me. In the last year or so of my pre-retirement life I spent an inordinate amount of time wondering if people were thinking I was too old. When my assistant brought a chair for me so that I wouldn't have to stand for several hours during a lengthy school program, I worried that the implication was that I was too old and feeble to stand throughout the proceedings rather than seeing it as simply a courteous act. I started noticing older colleagues and seeing how hard they seemed to be working at the same sorts of things—looking youthful, working longer and harder than others but being careful to never say they were tired, and walking purposefully and jauntily. It all is just so much work!

I soon realized there were few models or ground rules for professional women retiring in 2013. There aren't even good words to describe what we are going through. Terms like "transition" and "next phase" seem a bit stilted for everyday use. The word retirement calls up images that many of us are uncomfortable with. I was determined not to use the word "retired" because of the negative images it evoked for me. After all, the dictionary defines "to retire" unappealingly as "to withdraw" and "to go to bed." I knew I wasn't ready to disappear into a back room. But what to put in its place? At the end of my final school year amidst the heartwarming going-away parties in my honor, my colleagues and students took to saying I was "graduating." I found that an endearing idea, but it has its limits in describing my new status. The problem with words is that they can determine both attitudes and perceptions. To say I'm retired I believe creates an impression of who I am and the life I'm living that are inaccurate. But the question that I live with each day remains, **"Who am I now that I've taken this step and what kind of life do I want to live?"** The answer is—I don't know yet. I don't have answers, just a flood of conflicting emotions and unanswered questions mingling with moments of both optimism and dread.

To a certain degree what I, and so many other women across America, are facing is a new phenomenon. As we became adults and chose our life paths, for the first time women increasingly began to choose some form of career over being full-time mothers and home-makers. Many of our mothers didn't have careers so they didn't have the same issues at our age. But I, along with many others of my generation, were "children of the 60s." We found meaning and purpose in our careers. Many of us had the quaint idea that we could change the world. I was a social worker for Headstart, taught students with severe emotional problems, and headed a school for students with disabilities because I felt it was important and meaningful work. I believed in "saving the world one child at a time." But now, suddenly, I don't feel that I am making a difference anymore. So I am left with a hole in my life where I used to feel a burning sense of purpose.

I saw a photograph not too long ago that struck me as rather chilling in this regard. I was reading a news article about the appointment of a new president for a major educational institution who would be replacing the current woman president. The large color photograph showed the new top executive sitting at a conference table giving his inaugural speech. The people seated around him—I assume they were his board of directors—were gazing at him raptly, clearly hanging on his every word. I also saw an attractive, well-dressed woman seemingly in her 60s sitting in the front row of the audience. I knew that she was the retiring president. On closer examination, I saw that there was something "off" about her body language. Of all the people in the room she seemed tense and unhappy. She was hiding it beautifully behind a dignified posture but it was her hands that gave her away. She was smiling (although rather stiffly), but her hands were locked tightly in her lap, clasped so firmly that it was possible to see even in the media photograph that her knuckles were white. She gave the impression of someone who was doing her duty graciously and with dignity even though the situation was uncomfortable for her. To go from being the speaker at the head table, the center of everyone's attention, to not being seated at the table at all is difficult, even if one is prepared for the transition. It is not even a matter of whether the decision was yours or whether it was thrust upon you by others. In any case, you are faced with trying to define your new role and adjusting to your new reality appropriately and with dignity. It is not easy.

I recently read a comment by Jane Pauley from her book dealing with the same transitional life I'm writing about. She said that she believes that there won't be the need for books like ours in the future because this trail that women are now blazing will be a familiar, taken-for-granted life stage. Part of me believes this to be true. I admire how smoothly and smartly women who grew up and matured in a different era with other mindsets and expectations handle issues with which I and my friends struggled such as careers, motherhood, and partnering in marriage. Yet, in order for things to change to that extent, there will need to be a major shift in our ideas about identity and worth and value. If we continue to define ourselves primarily by what we do and how successful we are in that arena, I'm afraid what I am facing will not be very much different for women in the future. I sincerely hope I am wrong.

I have always been a planner and I put a lot of thought into what I would do upon retirement. I had an idea for a service that would continue helping children and families and, that to be honest, would also provide some replacement income. I developed a page on the Internet and I found myself immersed in the dotcom world. I felt like Alice in Wonderland, bewilderingly confronted with choices to "link this" and "post that" and trying to figure things out with the help of my 20-something Web designer. I also had become happily involved in some hobbies that I truly enjoyed, most notably pastel painting, a late-in-life discovery that I loved doing and was actually pretty good at. So I felt that I was prepared for this next stage in my life. I had made plans for something I could do that would keep me involved with the educational and advocacy issues I cared about, a family I loved and would be able to spend quality time with, and an artistic outlet that let me express my creative side.

So far, things have not worked out quite as planned. **"Rocky beginning"** rather than **"smooth sailing"** would more accurately describe what I'm going through. The best way to explain is that I feel as though I'm in a state of suspended animation. I'm not moving ahead—in fact I'm uncertain at this point as to which direction "ahead" would be. I'm questioning a number of the assumptions with which I entered this process. Self-doubt and lack of confidence—two things that have never characterized me—are creeping into my thinking, and, most troubling, I feel that right now I am living the life of "retirement" that I most feared.

I have never been a "quitter." I am better known as being doggedly determined and I am challenged and stimulated by solving problems. So—at least on good days—I believe I can figure this out. I know that it will take patience (another quality that has never characterized me), although I am also acutely aware that I don't have a whole lifetime of opportunities stretching ahead of me. The luxury of time has cushioned other transition points in my life, but now time is ticking away along with my options. No one who knows me believes that I will be content with doing nothing. "So what are you going to do next?" crops up at some point in almost every conversation with friends and family members as they repeat the same conviction that there must be something else for me to do and contribute. They all reassure me that I shouldn't worry because it will become clear what that is. The general agreement is that I'm not the kind of person to retire. I agree. I have always thought I was more the "don't go quietly into that good night" kind of person. But, I have no idea what that special thing is. I am beginning to entertain the possibility that there may be nothing to that. That who we **are** is not necessarily who we **were**. I may need to adjust to the reality that aging changes things and that I need to approach life with a different mindset. I have given myself time to figure out this transition and I am only in the first month, but I do want to be intentional about the journey if for no other reason than to pass on what I have learned to my own daughters and granddaughters. So I will continue to journal, to think, to have conversations with anyone who is willing to talk with me about how they are handling all this, and to struggle with my doubts, my worries, and my dreams. I do believe that it's all about the journey, no matter how daunting that journey might be.

So now I have a plan: to chronicle my retirement journey for one year. It started as my own personal journal of ups and downs, discoveries and insights. Then I began talking about my project and was somewhat surprised at how many of my friends and acquaintances admitted to being in the same situation. The common sentiment is pretty much that those of us in our 60s in 2014 are, to a great extent, entering uncharted waters without much in the way of patterns, mentors, or templates. We are capable, articulate and intelligent and yet we seem to have trouble clearly seeing the path ahead. As one friend said, "This whole idea of retiring is new for women in general. Men have been dealing with this for a long time—and often handling it badly." But this is new ground for us. I believe that we women can collectively figure out how to move on in our lives with grace and courage and joy. Women are communicators and empathizers and we are in this together. It doesn't even have to do with whether we had a full-time career or not. The fact that we are a transitional generation of women means that many more things are shifting under our feet than simply whether we still get up and go to work every morning. My friends who made the choice to raise their children and make things better in their communities as their career, find themselves in the middle of the same normlessness. They are dealing with things like the largely modern phenomenon of children and grandchildren moving hundreds of miles away and no longer being a regular part of their lives, or possibly the shifting of the valuable community work they have enjoyed doing through the years to other hands. Whether we have been career women in the traditional sense or not, we are all faced with decisions about what to do that will be meaningful and fulfilling in the years ahead.

So I have dedicated myself to this year of writing about my experiences for a two-fold reason. I need a catharsis, a way of organizing my thinking that helps me see more clearly and get some understanding of how to live my new reality. But I also love research—an affinity I acquired during the many years I have spent earning a variety of degrees. In my more objective, less emotionally involved moments, I look at this period with a researcher's eye. I wonder what we can learn about life after retirement and the possibilities as well as the pitfalls. Is there a body of wisdom out there, or ready to be developed, that can make the years ahead truly "The Golden Years?" Or is that phrase simply designed to convince us that we are enjoying something that we really are not.

In that spirit I am hoping you will join me as I chronicle this journey. The question for me is, whether there is hope that I, and in fact all of us, can come out of this wiser, stronger and more at peace? Instead of a time of diminishment and dwindling hopes and possibilities could these next years be a time of expansion and fulfillment? It is supremely important for me to find out. I deeply believe that as we share our stories we gather the strength and wisdom we need for our own lives. I know that's very true for me. In fact, it was a story told by a dear friend as we sat on her deck gazing at Lake Michigan that has been a continuing inspiration to me.

This friend is an intelligent, gracious woman who I would admire even if she weren't dealing so courageously with a serious, and rather rare, blood disease. She was at the height of her career, as a speech therapist working with young children when the disease hit. She had to end her successful practice and the consulting, speaking, and teaching that had made her a prominent voice in the field. However, she didn't retreat into self-pity but rather focused outward, reaching out to other women. When one of her close friends was diagnosed with breast cancer, they decided that they would meet once a week. They spread the word that any woman who was in a similar situation was welcome to join them. The only stipulation was that group members would take turns planning the meetings and whoever was in charge of planning had to come up with something that was just simply fun. They took field trips to out-of-the-way places, luxuriated with spa treatments, and one day they each bought a wildly decadent pair of shoes and then individually decorated them to make them even more unique. But there was also an understanding that each of these smart and capable women should not stop dreaming and that the group would never be a replacement for those dreams. When any one of them found something to become involved in that was personally important and meaningful to her, she should move on—the group would have served its purpose. As my friend told the story, some amazing friendships developed in that group of women and it was an incredibly important support for women going through rocky times. She went on to say the point came when she and her friend who had started the group were the only two women left. All the others had indeed found something to devote themselves to. There was joy in my friend's voice as she talked about the wonderful things that had come from that group of women who were there to give each other strength and the courage to step out and try something new. Interestingly, the co-founder of the group had a dream of wanting to open a knitting shop. My friend is an accomplished knitter so they decided to fulfill that dream by becoming partners in a small yarn store. Today they have a thriving business and my friend is happily conducting classes and sharing her wisdom and common sense with many other women just like she did with the 12 women in that special group—and me. As my friend completed her story she said, **"The thing is, women always find a way to come together and support each other—it's what we do."** I believe her

2

Every Journey Starts With a Single Step-- But In What Direction?

*"The best time to plant a tree was 20 years ago.
The next best time is now."*

— CHINESE PROVERB

I HAVE ALWAYS loved reading magazines and journals. One of my teen aged memories from the early 60's was learning with my friends what it meant to be a fashionable young woman through the pages of *Seventeen* magazine. We learned essential beauty tips such as how to roll our hair on orange juice cans to achieve a smooth, sophisticated hairdo and steps we could take to make us look more like Sandra Dee or Annette Funicello. I still read magazines every chance I get. Thoughtful commentary, political opinions, and information about parts of the world I don't spend enough time thinking about are all at my beck and call in their pages. As a self-taught artist, I have learned much from art journals featuring talented artists and their philosophies and techniques. One of the magazine columns I regularly read is Oprah's "What I Know for Sure." Every month Oprah shares an inspirational thought that she believes in enough to stake her confidence on. As I step out onto these new and unfamiliar paths and the flood of conflicting feelings that have been part of the last two months, I realize I will need a foundation—a bedrock of belief

I can use to anchor myself so I'm not just aimlessly wandering. So I decided to follow Oprah's lead and begin to decide what I really do believe that will direct me in this new life. It is not an easy assignment for an inherent skeptic, but after much reflection I came to the conclusion that, as a start, there are a few things I can hang my hat on that I believe about this next phase of my life. I don't always live them, but I do believe them.

I believe, in the quaint words made famous by a recent president known for his creative use of words that **"I am the Decider."** My circumstances will not ultimately determine my attitude if I don't let them. My outlook on life each day is my choice. I believe that if I am depressed or bitter I have given myself permission (which I sadly do more than I would like.) As Abraham Lincoln famously said, **"Most people are about as happy as they make up their minds to be."** So, even if nothing turns out to match the retirement scenario I have imagined, I have control over how I respond.

As I write this, I acknowledge that beliefs don't always translate into actions. And even when behavior is changed, those changes are not always sustained. We all have attended seminars and workshops when, inspired by dynamic speakers and energized by group enthusiasm, we walk out fired up and determined to make a change in some area of our lives. A few weeks or months later a pretty high percentage of us have returned to the old habits we fervently believed we had discarded. I do know, however, that if I am going to achieve authentic happiness and contentment in the coming years it will need to come from within me. If I am the "Decider" then it is my choice if I allow myself to feel invisible and stuck in the suspended animation state I wrote about last month. It is a tall order, but I don't see any way around it.

Another thing I am sure about is that a primary source of those positive feelings is to find what makes me happy and do it. That is where the Chinese proverb I quoted at the beginning of this section comes in. In addition to sharing what she believes to be true, Oprah has a consistent message about living our best lives, lives that are not only happy, but that have meaning and purpose. At this stage we can't afford to put off finding what we are passionate about and doing it. I know for sure that days are passing and they are precious and I want to live them fully and joyfully.

All these things sound so easy and self-evident. If I want to be happy I need to cultivate a positive attitude that accepts my present life with both its gifts and losses, finding the silver lining in the losses and accepting the gifts with gratitude. It also makes complete sense that I will be more fulfilled if I am doing what I love to do and if what I love to do has meaning for me. I can say that all of this I believe. But there is a fine balance there. I also believe that finding out what gives me happiness and what is meaningful for me requires a level of self-knowledge that will come only as I take time to think and reflect. I envision that it will be hard work or else I would already be confidently sailing into the future doing what I love to do. I read somewhere that getting to know ourselves is a lifetime job. I am ready to get started. I will feel far better if I plant that long-put-off tree than if I sit around feeling sorry for myself.

Since I started this section with Oprah's words I will end with them as I quote, **"Your journey begins with a choice, to get up, step out, and live fully."** That sounds like the direction I would like to be heading and I am hopeful.

3

Who Am I Really?

"It's never too late to be what you might have been."

— GEORGE ELIOT

"I AM AN artist." I'm practicing saying this with pride. At first it was hard to say for two reasons. First, because it was so improbable. I have always enjoyed looking at good art and visiting art galleries yet I have never had the slightest interest in creating my own art until two years ago. The second stumbling block to saying I am an artist is that it sounds boastful to me. I don't know why this is true since I've never had a problem with saying that I am a teacher or a Head of School. In fact I've never had much trouble saying "I'm an excellent teacher," but proclaiming that I'm an artist seems to be perplexingly in a different category. It seems to be more presumptive. It falls into the same category as saying "I'm pretty" because being an artist has the connotation of a natural "gift" that sets one apart rather than something one works at and grows into. At any rate, whatever my feelings are about saying it, I am learning to feel comfortable with it. My comfort level got a boost when former president George W. Bush said about his post-retirement discovery of oil painting, "**I've discovered I have a Rembrandt inside me.**" That's what I call confidence.

In my last entry I challenged myself to find something that made me happy and do it. I am in a really good place right now having come to the realization that I can do what I really love to do and feel good about it rather than feeling guilty because I'm not doing something more serious, significant and worthwhile. The service I created that counsels parents in the development of their child's IEP (Individualized Educational Plan) to make sure that their child has the best educational opportunities has never gotten off the ground. There seem to be a number of reasons for it, but among them are that, regardless of the claims of my young "techie" friends, there are still services that do not work well online.. This business plan of mine seems to be one of them. Parents want help dealing with the complexities of special education, but they really want face-to-face help. I completely understand that. Entrusting their child's educational future to someone they have never met is risky. People do call me for advice and I am happy to answer their questions. I love helping them, but I am uncomfortable charging for that help. So, it's clear that it really isn't a business—at least at this point. It's also clear that I am an educator but probably not a businessperson. The interesting part is that when I came to the realization that my planned venture was not working, I was a bit regretful, but I wasn't terribly sad. This brings me back to the statement I started this section with: "I am an artist." I think my business plan was a false start because it was based on the belief that I should stick with what I have always done in defining the work I should do in this next stage. I have been an educator all my professional life and education is the world in which I move most comfortably. Hence, it seemed to make sense to use what I know in discovering my new direction. That seems to many of us to be a reasonable assumption. Surely the knowledge and experience gained in a particular field should be valuable and—yes—marketable. Yet in the professional world where people are slotted into positions and traditional thinking is the norm, it is not always easy to see where we fit.

I haven't totally thrown in the towel. I may return to delivering that service at some point if I develop greater clarity as to how it could work. I absolutely believe in the importance of making sure disabled children have the very best educational plan in place and I also believe that it is a complex process and many parents need expert help in making that happen. However, I also agree with the wise saying, **"If you don't know what to do, do nothing."** So, for now I will do what I love to do —my pastel painting and just wait to see what might happen with my IEP service in the future. For right now I am happiest and most peaceful when I am creating a painting. I love planning my next project when I am down and want to feel better. Once I made that discovery, I have also realized that I can give myself permission to do what I enjoy. That may not sound like a revolutionary discovery to many of you, but to someone like me who has a strong sense of obligation and duty combined with a feeling that I should devote myself only to serious and meaningful endeavors, this idea was indeed novel…and incredibly freeing. I was extremely interested to find that science affirms the benefits of this idea. It even has its own theory—**self-affirmation theory.** According to Geoffrey Cohen, a noted social psychologist and researcher, affirming oneself in a whole new, unrelated domain is a powerful way to restore self-esteem. So it's healthy for me to say loud and clear: "I am an artist!" I challenge you to try this in an area that is new and fresh for you. It truly does feel good.

I believe I am now ready to say "yes" to re-imagining myself. I feel like a whole new life awaits me! I have started thinking about ways to market my art although I am also feeling freed—at least somewhat—from my belief that I must make money to help support our retirement lifestyle. I am still serious about contributing to our finances and I am not comfortable simply being one of the "ladies who do lunch" without a thought to the future. But I am now of the mind that bringing in money should **follow** the joy, rather than **being** the joy.

As confirmation of my new direction I actually sold a painting! The buyer is a friend, but, in my elation, I am convinced he would have bought it anyway. I'm excited and believe that I am on the right path. I expect that there will be bumps in the road, but I am—at least for now—at peace.

4

The Best-Laid Plans

"We are not human beings having a spiritual experience, we are spiritual beings having a human experience"

— Pierre Teilhard de Chardin

MY THANKS GO to Oprah for sharing the above quote. I admire Oprah. I like her spirit and her smartness and her words frequently inspire me. I also am an avid saver of quotes. I love mulling over words that speak to me and when I come across a particularly meaningful thought I make sure to put it in my journal to remember it and be inspired by it. I must admit though that, at first, although I did find de Chardin's words intriguing, it wasn't one of those sayings that immediately grabbed me and spoke to me. But for some reason I wrote his words down and I can't get them out of my mind. I am now beginning to see why.

On December 20 everything changed for me. My new found peace and sense of direction were shattered. My husband and I were in the midst of our usual hectic holiday plans. We have 5 children and 5 grandchildren who live in various far-flung places, so Christmas planning is generally a juggling act. For the past few years our routine has been to drive to Northern Indiana to share Christmas Eve and several days leading up to it with our two daughters and sons-in-law and their children: our eldest granddaughter, Ana, her 4-year old brother Nate, and the adorable baby and youngest grandchild, Elle who, as the youngest, is the "star of the show." Then we fly to California on Christmas day to be with our eldest son, his wife and two other special granddaughters, Campbell and Lauren, in Marin County. I had spent the day of December 20 buying ingredients for home made Christmas cookies. I was excited that I would have the time to bake for the first time in several years and I had thrown myself into the nostalgia of collecting cookie recipes my mother, mother-in-law and old friends had used. I had also been running around buying last minute gifts. I had not taken the time to eat all day and, in addition, my doctor had been experimenting with different dosages of blood pressure medicine. As a result of all that I began to feel light headed and went outside to get some fresh air. I fainted and fell down a flight of brick steps outside our back door. It was a horrible accident that resulted in my being rushed by ambulance to the local hospital trauma center. I left the trauma center two days later after receiving 28 stitches in my head and a cast for a right wrist that had been broken in two places. I also had a broken bone under my eye, a concussion, and a severely bruised hip that is excruciatingly painful. Suddenly, as a result of one 5-minute incident, I found myself in a physical and psychological pit and sinking fast. I walk haltingly with a cane that prevents me from my new conscientious determination to exercise more regularly and has forced me, at least temporarily, into a sedentary life style that is depressing under any circumstances. I ache all over and feel helpless as I have found how difficult and cumbersome it is to try to function with a broken right wrist when one is right handed. But, most of all, I feel overcome by the one thing I most feared and wanted to avoid—I feel old!

My lowest point came in a conversation with my 9-year old granddaughter, Ana, one day when I was struggling to navigate with my cane. There are a number of family jokes about how much we are alike and she looks up to me and is proud to be "just like Nana." This matters greatly to me and I very much want to be a good example and mentor for her. On this particular occasion she said, "Nana, I can help you. You have to be careful because you're fragile." **Fragile?!** I have always prided myself on being strong and determined and now my beloved granddaughter thinks I'm fragile!

Recently I have returned to the words of Teilhard de Chardin and I have begun reflecting on his thinking on our spirituality in light of all that has happened. I am not an overtly religious person, but I do believe there are things at work in the world—spiritual principles—that are beyond my understanding. I have seen what I believe to be karma at work in the events of my life and the lives of others I know and I believe that putting good out into the universe has strong and beautiful results. So it seems so sadly ironic that just as I believed that I had things figured out and my forward path was clear, everything seemed to crash around me. It is even more ironic that I broke my right wrist, rendering me unable to paint, so soon after my triumphant statement claiming that "I am an artist." Is there something going on at a spiritual level that I don't understand? How large a part has my unconscious played in what has happened? All of these questions and dark thoughts swirl around in my brain as I see the exciting journey into the next phase of my life derailed and lying in ruins around me.

Although I do believe that sometimes bad things do just happen and that not everything always happens for a purpose (or at least a purpose we can understand,) I have been wondering recently if there is something I can learn from this miserable turn of events. In reflecting on this one day I turned to my husband and asked, "Do you think that accident would have happened if I hadn't retired?" I do know that there is a solid body of research into the connection between our mental state and our physical wellbeing. Could there be an equally strong connection between our mental state and actions that we take that can cause accidents? Maybe there is something deeper going on that I should pay attention to and learn from. I believe there is a possibility that I have been so busy moving forward and "figuring things out" that it would take something pretty major to catch my attention. I also think that where we are mentally and emotionally can be a risk factor. I certainly don't mean that I subconsciously brought about my fall through suppressed self-destructive urges. That's not what I'm saying at all. But I do think that it's extremely possible that one's mental state—sadness, discouragement, isolation—is a major factor in how our lives play out. Possibly the problem with our unconscious thoughts is that without even realizing it, we get the notion that we aren't really that important or worthy anymore, so we don't take care of ourselves as well as we should. This, then, can combine with a low-level depressed state to make us less healthy and more accident-prone. I realize that I need to include social connectedness, fun, healthy eating, and exercise in my new life plan.

When I was younger I was a night owl and somewhat of a stress addict with a lifestyle fueled by lots of coffee and something quick and easy eaten on the run for lunch. But now, all that has to change and I need to be very mindful and intentional about how I take care of my health. It may additionally be true that things haven't been as '"settled" and happily optimistic as I had thought. Possibly my feelings just went underground and I still have some learning and growing to do. Maybe there is more to the reality of our spiritual sides than we realize. I don't know if there's anything to these reflections, but I am open to the possibility.

However, I don't want to wallow in self-pity. Things are looking up. As I resume writing this after a couple of weeks I am starting to feel better, the cane is gone, healing is progressing nicely, my doctors all say I am lucky, and I learned some pretty important lessons.

I also have developed a new and unexpected skill that has both lifted my spirits and been personally quite meaningful to me. Aside from the pain and inconvenience of all of this, my biggest disappointment was that my newfound life in art had come to a screeching halt before it even had the opportunity to get off the ground. Then one morning soon after the accident happened I was on a long-distance call with my son Chris when he asked me an interesting question. He wondered if I would be able to paint with my pastels held in my left hand? I gave it a try and, amazingly enough, it turned out much better then I had imagined it would. I was flabbergasted! Not only did it work, it actually worked smoothly and easily. It felt so natural that I found myself not even giving a thought to which hand I was using. This must be what Csikszentmihalyi means by "being in the flow." I have never had even a hint that I could be ambidextrous in any way. That certainly didn't change since I have had to sign some things recently with my left hand and my left-handed writing is illegible and horribly shaky. But, strangely, I can actually paint with my left hand almost as well as with my right. Since then I have heard that some artists recommend practicing painting with one's opposite hand because it can loosen up the movements and make a more flowing painting. That sounds good to me since loosening up and relinquishing tight control is what a lot of this journey is all about. This has meant a great deal to me as I can still do what I love. But even more importantly, I have been able to show my granddaughter, Ana, lessons about perseverance, determination, and starting over. Recently I was talking with my two daughters and Ana about downsizing and the conversation moved into what sentimental objects they would like to have. I was touched when Ana spoke up and said that the one thing she would want to have is one of my left-handed pastels. It makes up for the "fragile" remark and brings to mind a wise statement about turning lemons into lemonade.

> *Note: A few days ago I was watching a golf tournament on television and the announcer said that Phil Mickelson is actually right handed even though he golfs with his left hand. It's pretty cool having this in common with one of the world's top golfers. It would be even better if I could be as successful as he has been with this quirky little talent! On the off chance that*

there is something here, I am now signing the paintings that I do with my left hand in the left corner instead of my normal right corner. It's good to be prepared!

I was determined to still go to California. I knew how much my granddaughters, Campbell and Lauren have been looking forward to the visit, and I knew how terribly disappointed I would be not to see them. I had to schedule follow-up appointments with all the doctors who had seen me in the hospital, but my husband finally agreed that if I received permission from the doctors, we would reschedule. So, on New Year's Day instead of Christmas Day we were on the plane for Northern California.

I'm sad that Campbell and Lauren live too far away to allow me to spend as much time with them as I would like, but they visit us each summer for an extended time in Michigan and we visit them at Christmas. Now that I am retired I plan on having more opportunities to enjoy these little girls. Campbell is 5 years old and is in kindergarten. I am sure her kindergarten teacher wishes there were more of Campbell since she is a sweet-natured child who loves school, works hard to do her best, and is generous and kind. She also **loves** art. Her mother, Julie, does amazing things with crafts so Campbell calls us the "three girl artists." When I am with her we spend hours doing art together and it is a special bond between us. Lauren is mischievous and tremendously funny. She is a free spirit who loves nothing better then to put on one of her costumes and launch into an interpretive dance.

The whole thing about grandchildren is mystifying to me. Friends have been telling me for years about the joys of being a grandparent, but I was skeptical. Many of these same friends fondly remember the years when they stayed home with toddlers as the happiest years of their life and they even claimed that the teenaged years weren't so bad! Clearly we inhabited a different reality. But they were right about grandchildren. I am now as prone as any other grandmother to bore anyone who will listen with endless stories illustrating my grandchildren's cuteness and superior intelligence, something I found reprehensible until it became my turn. It amazes me that these interesting, beautiful, wise little people actually love to spend time with me. And the best part is how much I enjoy being with them. They make me laugh and sometimes cry and it's a privilege to be part of their lives. They can also bring us to see ourselves in a different light and teach us important lessons. Campbell showed me that I needed to rethink one of my most cherished assumptions and, in the process, question a belief I have held for many years.

One of the guiding principles of my life has been the importance of setting an example for my daughters of what women can accomplish. Whatever I have done in my adult life I believed had the added impetus of showing my two girls that women can be strong and do whatever they want to do. That was not the model that was set for me growing up in the 50s and 60s when it was common knowledge that men would go out in the world and accomplish things while a woman's place was in the home. I cheer Sheryl Sandberg when she says that boys who dominate are called leaders while girls are called "bossy." I was called "bossy" on many occasions and I wanted to pass on a different heritage to my daughters. It troubles me that the clearest memory of me that my granddaughters will have is that of being retired. They will not remember when I was involved in my career or taking the plunge to live in an apartment in New York city by myself for a year so I could teach at Teacher's College, Columbia University thrilled to follow in the footsteps of educational giants like John Dewey. I won't be able to share with them the experience of walking across the stage to accept my doctorate degree. But, as I learned from Campbell, there may be other lessons that are even more important.

I had great times on our visit to California reading stories and playing cards with "Lauren the card shark and Uno Master" and, of course, doing art with Campbell. She was beside herself with excitement to give me her very special Christmas present, a session at a local art and ceramics studio to make an art piece together. She kept asking with her eyes sparkling if I loved my present. Every day included an art session with the "girl artists." I amazed everyone with my left-handed prowess. Then one day Campbell said an odd thing. In a quiet voice she asked if I would do a really bad painting. Not quite understanding why, I did what she asked and we laughed about it as we took turns adding features that made it even more ugly and grotesque. It became clear to me by some of her comments as we worked on the really ugly painting that she had been feeling diminished as she compared her art to mine. I remembered back to the number of times she had said, "Oh Nana, yours is so good and mine's so bad." I also remembered even further back to a few times when one of my daughters said something similar like, "Oh Mom, I could never do what you do." Of course they are wrong. We each have gifts and talents and one person's achievement is not another's and certainly it is silly to even consider comparing the drawing of a 5 year old with that of a grown woman. But maybe all of the effort I had put into making sure my daughters and granddaughters got the message about achievement and their limitless potential and possibilities had backfired a bit. Maybe it is every bit as important for them to see the reality of the number of times I fail with the lesson being how that failure is handled. It was an amazing revelation to me, and very freeing, to realize that an ugly drawing by her Nana may be just what my little granddaughter needed to gain confidence in her **own** gifts and talents. The most valuable mentoring I may accomplish for my family could be to fail, then share with them honestly and openly how I feel, and finally pick myself up and go on. I certainly have the opportunity to do that where I am now!

The positive side of failure has been getting quite a lot of press recently. The part failing plays in learning and growing and giving us the unsought-for, but valuable, opportunity to re-imagine ourselves is being increasingly explored. In addition there is the thought that if we haven't failed, we may have been playing it too safe. In a recent interview after a tournament marked by shots that went wild followed by amazing saves out of bunkers, my favorite "left-handed golfer," Phil Mickelson said, **"A safe shot is when you don't have the nerve to take a risk."** I am coming to the realization that I would rather aim high and miss than play it safe.

Jane Pauley said in her book that one of the greatest gifts she gave her children was failing at her daytime show. She explained that, **"From a distance it looks like I had one success after another and I think that's how my children looked at my career until that show failed."** It is a surprising idea for me. I have always been able to see the strength in surviving times when things fell apart with your head held high. In fact, another one of my favorite quotes to live by has been **"Whatever doesn't kill you makes you stronger."** (As an aside, my daughters have a pure hatred for that quote as would any teen aged girl whose mother remorselessly repeated those words each time her world was falling apart and her heart was broken.) But this is different. It's not so much gutting through or being tough and "showing people what you're made of." This is saying that failing can actually be a gift. And, even more, it is not just a gift to you in your own personal growth. It is a gift you can give to your children who are watching you and learning from you about humility and honesty and resilience. As Brene Brown, author and speaker who identifies herself as a vulnerability researcher puts it, the important thing is **"Showing up, taking risks, and letting myself be seen."** I'm starting to become excited about being free enough to let those I love see me with all my flaws and missteps and fears.

My final thought on this subject is actually a question I have begun asking myself lately: **"What is it I am aiming for and what risks are worth taking?"** If I take these words to heart and go charging off in the direction of proving myself once again, the danger is that I will be back to the lifestyle of striving and overworking that I have led all my life. One of the lessons I believe all this has been teaching me is that much of my angst and unhappiness in the time immediately following my retirement was a result of pride and the fear of what other people were thinking—or not thinking—about me. I find words like "I feel invisible" and "I'm not making a difference anymore" quite revealing because these statements are very other-directed. Other people's opinions determine those feelings. So, aiming high for me might very well be seeking inner peace and a different kind of joy. Maybe the example is how to deal with the different "times and seasons" in my life with grace and happiness and yet continue to make a difference in new and interesting ways rather than continuing to beat that proverbial dead horse. Demonstrating a life well lived in retirement is what I am aiming for. Now I just have to figure that out.

5

Taking Stock

*"If you can't fly then run,
If you can't run then walk,
If you can't walk then crawl,
But whatever you do, you have
to keep moving forward."*

— Martin Luther King, Jr.

I HAVE ALMOST reached the halfway mark of my "Year of Discovery" and I'm not sure how to gauge where I am in the journey. I have discovered a new talent and even sold a painting, I have been asked to present some workshops in a school district near our home in Northern Michigan and that is encouraging. I have had a life-changing accident and made it through.

Having the luxury of time to reflect and question, the main conclusion I have reached is that change is unavoidable no matter how hard we try to control our lives. What we can control is the direction that change takes us. The question in my mind at this half-way point is, what are the lessons that I have learned and how can I use them? I am still learning. First of all, when I say "lessons learned" I should in truth say "lessons I am learning…and relearning" This is much like the AA philosophy through which members are careful to say that they are "recovering" not "recovered." There are certain truths that have presented themselves to me and I have been given the opportunity (or challenge) to continue to work on learning the lessons they present every day.

I am learning to be patient both with myself and with the process I am going through. The initial period of angst and unhappiness when I first retired was largely the result of my expectations. I expected that I would immediately begin an exciting new phase of life, moving seamlessly into my next challenging and successful venture, whatever that would be. When the constantly ringing phone became much more quiet and the number of emails that crowded my inbox dropped off dramatically, I realized that people were moving on without feeling the need to seek my advice and wisdom. I couldn't believe how quickly that happened! I felt self-reproach as I woke up every morning with renewed determination to come up with a momentous plan that would fill my emptiness and then reached evening having procrastinated through another day. I felt like a failure. I had bought into the admiring and encouraging words of my friends and colleagues that with my wisdom and experience in the field of education, I would be in so much demand my problem would be that I would be too busy. I believed that would indeed be the case and yet I found I was wrong—or at least that it wasn't going to happen immediately. I no longer had a position of power. Now I am starting to see a difference. I still feel impatient at times, but things are starting to gradually fall into place and my attitude is much more calm and accepting of the reality of my life. I don't mean to give the impression that I'm sitting in a chair doing nothing but "relaxing" or that I don't care anymore. I am far from being retired in that sense of the word. I still want to be vital and involved in things that are engaging and challenging. I still wake up in the morning with plans to pursue. But I have shifted my idea of what constitutes time well spent. I am finding that I don't have to depend on my reputation and influence to feel a sense of accomplishment. I don't have to rush from project to project to prove I am important. I am finding enjoyment in personally rewarding pursuits like writing and painting. It is my hope that my writing might make a difference, but that's not my sole purpose in doing it. I am writing because I have things I want to say and ideas I want to share with whoever is interested. I still believe that there is a way for me to actively contribute and be involved, but I have become willing to accept that I need to watch and wait and expect that when the time is right I will know it.

I am learning (and sometimes it has been a hard lesson) to take better care of myself. Seeing the horrifying effect my accident had on my family, how deeply it frightened and saddened them, made an indelible impression on me. We owe it, not only to ourselves, but to our loved ones, to guard our health. As much as I dread feeling and looking old, being chauffeured through the airport in a wheelchair and walking with great pain leaning on a cane certainly did not help with my desire for a youthful image. I am learning that I must pay as much attention to my emotional needs as my physical ones. I never really gave these things much thought before. I was too busy. Happiness, health, and wellbeing were on the back burner way behind accomplishment. I want to use my time now to nourish my spirit and my body. I want to spend time with good friends; read good books; be open to new experiences and adventures; keep up with current events and new ideas; and be curious and interested. Certainly when I think about lessons to pass on to my children and grandchildren, a peaceful, generous spirit; an active, open mind; and being healthy enough to spend active time with them rank right at the top.

In addition to taking care of my physical and mental health, I have thought a great deal lately about **attitude.** When I "people watch" at public places, I tend to zero in on the older people in the crowd because of where I am in my life. One of my first impressions of many of the older people I see is that they too frequently look unhappy and grim. They send out vibes that somehow life has not turned out the way they had hoped and they are bitter about it. I don't want that to be me. I want to have a good sense of humor and be someone people feel comfortable talking to. I also want to be careful about sharing my "wisdom" (i.e. judgments that older people think everyone needs to hear and that can tend to be harsh and sharp-tongued). At base, I want to be open to all the ways life **has** turned out the way I had hoped and be **grateful.**

I am also learning the importance of trying new things and taking chances. I have talked about the great joy I am finding in my pastel painting. That has been the best thing about retirement. It is not just the painting. It is the pleasure of feeling comfortable and free to do something I really want to do when—and how often—I want to do it without the pressing sense of guilt that I have felt most of my life whenever I spend too much time on "leisure" activities or "hobbies." I am pretty sure I speak for many of us when I say that we have a strong sense of what constitutes a worthwhile use of time. Work is in a far different category from play. Many of us grew up with the rule of thumb that is frequently called "Grandma's Law"—you must eat your vegetables before you can have dessert. So we feel rather guilty and indulgent if we spend too much time just doing something enjoyable. When I first started allowing myself to feel okay about spending time doing what gave me pleasure, I was surprised at the number of times I caught myself at the end of the day saying that I had done nothing when in actuality I had spent a delightful afternoon in my art studio. Once I realized my time is my own and I don't need to justify how I spend it, I have discovered there are a number of other things I am interested in as well. I spent an entire day playing with clay with Campbell. We created a family and every kind of animal we could think of to go with them. I had so much fun, I have entertained thoughts of actually buying my own clay. I'm sure many of us as adults could benefit from the soothing activity of kneading clay. Recently, I found a book containing a daily lesson exploring creativity with water colors. I bought my supplies and am giving that a try. In addition, I have a number of subjects, like trying to understand the environment and global warning, that I would like to research. My goal would not be to produce a scholarly document or journal article but just to learn. Most importantly, I would like to volunteer my time and abilities to a meaningful cause. I will have more to say on that later.

Finally, I am learning how to live comfortably with my imperfections, my fallibility and my failures. I am practicing not taking myself too seriously and being able to laugh at myself and my foibles and faux pas. I want to develop a positive attitude and a kind spirit. Being understanding and forgiving of myself and those I love is my goal.

With all these lessons I'm working on, I figure my plate is pretty full. But something keeps coming up that makes me realize there are still some loose ends and I have not quite figured things out yet. We aren't settled on where we should live. When I retired, our goal was to relocate to our home in Michigan and that would be our principal residence. It's a lovely home nestled in the dunes with a gorgeous view and a beach on Lake Michigan. As I drew close to my retirement date we began moving more and more of our belongings up North. We stayed in Michigan from June until the end of October with an occasional foray back home for appointments. We made a number of discoveries during those months. We found that we love it in the fall. We would not be anywhere else. We could stroll the beach in solitude and the fall leaves were spectacular. But we made another discovery. Starting at the end of October we were quite isolated. To put it simply, we were a bit lonely. The peace and solitude that were so welcome when it was a retreat from our busy lives became awfully quiet when it was that way all the time. The closer it gets to November, the fewer people remain until we reach the point that we look out of our windows at night and our commanding view of the bay shows pure blackness. We have mixed feelings about the fact that ours are the only lights on in the entire vicinity. There are occasional get-togethers when all of us remaining in the surrounding area (all 20 or so of us) get together for a perch dinner at the only local restaurant that stays open into November. With the fall of the first snowflakes we watch the last of the "part-timers" pack up their cars for warmer climes and we fight the temptation to think of them as deserters.

We were among those who left at the beginning of November for our family Christmas activities planning to return in January in time for me to conduct the first of my school workshops. We returned as scheduled although we were hesitant due both to my injuries and the fact that this winter has shaped up to be by far the coldest and snowiest winter the Midwest has seen in years. Although we did not realize it, on our first winter day at our Michigan home we would be in for an experience that raised some questions about where we would be living our retirement life.

We pulled out of our driveway heading for my workshop for school paraprofessionals in a town about 30 miles away. I was looking forward to my first official foray back into the educational world since leaving Midwest Academy. My husband had decided to drive me there because it was starting to snow and I still have a cast on my wrist and need a cane to navigate. I know the following experience sounds odd, but you need to know that Northern Michigan weather is known for dramatic changes and improbable occurrences. When we left our home and headed down our steep driveway that extends from the top of our dune to the road, a moderately light snow instantly changed to something that looked uncomfortably like a blizzard. The wind had been picking up all morning and blowing snow into drifts and as we drove down our lane the wind rapidly created a serious white out condition. Our car became stuck in a snowdrift and we were surrounded by a wall of white. Snow piled up against the car doors and soon we were unable to open them. We could only see the vaguest outline of pine trees that we knew to be no more than 10 feet ahead of us. Fortunately, we were able to call the man who plows our drive. I sat in the car impatiently waiting for him to make his way to us through the driving snow as the time for the workshop drew ever closer…and closer. Our friend arrived to pull us out and it turned out to be an impossible task. He broke 2 tow-ropes and yet wasn't able to budge us. The frigid north wind was blowing ever colder, the temperature was way below zero, and all we could see was a white wall surrounding us. I called the school district to set up a Skype conference, but when we tried to leave the car and climb the dune to our home to reach the computer, that too proved impossible. The snow was drifted waist high in places and our hands and faces were painfully wind whipped when we attempted to trudge only a few feet. We climbed back into the car to wait staring bleakly at a wall of snow as the excavators went to get a heavier truck. Finally, after 4 hours of sitting in the car, we were able to return to our home. I completely missed the workshop. The whole experience was a red flag when we consider living up north in the wintertime. We have been here for several winter weeks now and there are certainly positives to being here. It is gorgeous with pristine snow mounded on the dunes, the frozen lake, and ice-covered pine trees. The stillness is majestic. It is cozy and quiet and very conducive to writing, reading good books, painting, and having pleasant conversations in front of the fire. We have fallen into a comfortable routine. However, it is worrisome to think about what we would have done if that Friday trip had been a medical emergency. We would have been unable to get to the nearest hospital that even in good weather is an hour away. Being caught without groceries or other supplies is another worry as the closest grocery store is a half hour drive. The solitude is magnificent. The inability to easily access life's necessities can be a problem.

Slogging through waist-high snowdrifts and spending hours stranded in a car are not common problems among retirees, but there is another issue we are dealing with that tends to be a more familiar issue. That issue has to do with where one lives and what that means in terms of connectedness and defining the elements of a full and meaningful life. One of the positive incentives for me to retire was that it would give us the freedom to choose where to spend our time without that decision being dictated by my job. We were so looking forward to being free to spend those gloomy, slushy winter months in a warm climate where we could live a much healthier and happier lifestyle, soaking up the sun and getting plenty of exercise and fresh air. Then back to Michigan in the glorious summer and fall. Perfect. Unfortunately, it hasn't quite worked out as we had expected. We are finding that, this year at least, we feel like perpetual tourists. Our doctors and others who help us manage our lives are all in Indianapolis. Since we do have some health issues that require attention, we are in and out of Indianapolis regularly for appointments. We also still have a home there. We spend the bulk of our time in Michigan, but we are finding that Michigan in the dead of winter may not be the most practical location for us. We have complained bitterly about the dreary Midwest winters for years and yet, somewhat oddly, when we are finally able to go elsewhere, we're not sure where that would be. Should we sell our residence in Indiana and relocate to Michigan altogether? Possibly. But our daughter, son-in-law, and our adorable little granddaughter Elle are there and we truly enjoy spending time with them and being part of our granddaughter's life as she grows. We feel inundated by decisions and there are no clear answers. The second problem is a greater issue for us. We are starting to get the uncomfortable feeling that if we have a lifestyle of touching down temporarily in several places without sinking roots in any special place, we will not live the life of meaning and purpose we had dreamed of. Without ties to the community, friends that we spend time with regularly, and worthwhile activities that we enjoy, we fear that we will be missing out on an important dimension of what makes life full. Putting down roots is important if for no other reason than that we can get involved in things that matter to us and we are able to sustain that involvement over time. We feel a desire to become more connected to Harbor Springs, the attractive, forward-thinking little town near our Michigan home. But to do that requires that we commit to being there on a regular bases. I have had many thoughts of joining an art group, doing volunteer work, working with a school or teaching a class. But all of those things require being somewhere for a period of time. Right now I feel like we are in somewhat of a vicious cycle. I don't want to be a perpetual traveler, floating aimlessly with no meaningful ties to any community.

When I mentioned this dilemma of place and permanency over lunch with a dear friend, she gave me a different perspective to think about. As she pointed out, most of our friends are at the same place in life and are dealing with the same questions. If I made the decision to remain rooted in the community I have been part of for years for the purpose of maintaining connections, those special people I want to stay connected with will very possibly not be here all the time either. We are all pretty much in the same boat. So maybe, she suggested, the idea of community needs to have a different connotation for us. Possibly meeting somewhere for a special retreat or finding a way to mark and share special memories and occasions with those we care about will be part of developing a new way to be together. It is certainly something to think about.

6

Revisiting That Spiritual/Human Connection

> Beginnings
> In a human life, an infinite number
> of beginnings occur.
> I think beginnings are beautiful.
> They are a sign of hope and change.
> In the beginning, you have a renewed
> excitement for life.
> I believe the beginning is where magic is birthed.
>
> — Mindy Lacefield

IT IS ALWAYS in the night when it happens. I wake up with an almost physical feeling of emptiness and deep sadness. I feel a heavy sense of dread about my life, how little is remaining, and where it is heading as I lay in the darkness. During the day I am mostly happy and optimistic. But at 2:00 AM I can be blindsided. I also am aware that these times happen more frequently whenever it is time to return to our home in Indiana with its ties to my former life. I assume this always happens at those times because my defenses are down. I am happy that it doesn't happen more often because it is a truly miserable feeling. But I also feel that it is a wake up call, a small, psychic alarm in the darkness of the night reaching out to me precisely because that is when I am vulnerable and alone. I dread those moments and yet I am beginning to again think much more deeply and reflectively about myself as that "spiritual being who is having a human experience" that de Chardin speaks about. And I wonder what that means for me. Is the outer person I have always presented to the world in the process of falling away like clothes that don't fit anymore? Is there a more authentic and peaceful inner person waiting to step forward? I recently read some words from Brene Brown's most recent book that, although they sound deceptively simple, were incredibly meaningful to me. She talks about **the power to create and live by our own definitions.** Those are powerful words for someone like me. I believe, and have been told, that I give the impression of being an independent and strong woman who follows my own path and finds it quite easy to push on past what people think of me. That is not entirely accurate. It is true that I am determined and pretty relentless when it comes to something that matters to me. I am a "doer" with a strong backbone and plenty of confidence. But those characteristics live side-by-side in my psyche with a little girl who seeks approval and thrives on admiration. If I am feeling good about my accomplishments and the direction I am taking, I am quite able to attribute other people's negative comments to misunderstanding or envy or small-mindedness. However, if I am feeling insecure or unappreciated, I too easily try to win back the esteem and approval of others by allowing their priorities to set my agenda. So I have spent a lifetime with an internalized idea decided by society's conventions of what matters, what defines success for me, and how I measure up. I don't think I am unusual in this. I think most of us have lived our lives with much this same mindset.

If I am able to truly believe that I am primarily a spiritual being, then what I accomplish or who is impressed by what I do becomes less important than who I truly am. The internal me is what counts. To resist having my ideas of success and worth defined by everyone else "out there" and to be able to live by standards that I have chosen and believe in sounds wonderful. I still have some time here in this silent, snow-covered Michigan world to dig into this. This slow-paced environment certainly lends itself to the contemplative time I will need to get in touch with a meaningful sense of what I would define as the elements of a valuable and worthwhile life.

I am committing to this endeavor as of today: February 12, 2014. As I write this date I realize that Valentine's Day is two days away. I can't think of a better Valentine present to give myself than to free myself to live my life on my own terms with my own definitions of happiness, value, and success. Can I change enough at my age to be able to be able to think in terms of "being" instead of "doing?" I don't know, but I would like to try. I really don't have much choice at this point as I would be hard put to define myself in terms of what I do. I'm not doing much of anything that is definable. The path to happiness and inner peace in the upcoming years seems to be through focusing fully on who I am becoming. I don't think when De Charden speaks of us as spiritual beings, he is referring to a monastic retreat from the world. Having a human experience would surely include being involved in the things around us. But then the question remains: involved with who, where and in what way?

7

Forward Momentum in a Positive Direction

"The only real voyage of discovery consists not in seeking new landscapes, but in having new eyes."

— MARCEL PROUST

I AM WRITING this from our home in Indiana. We left Michigan last week and returned to our long-time community to attend to appointments and other mundane practicalities. The weather hasn't changed. We're approaching March and it's still bitterly cold and snowy. Choosing the coldest and most miserable Midwest winter in recent history to launch my post-retirement life hasn't made the transition any smoother. But something has changed within me. It started when we were in Michigan and is still continuing. It can best be described as a sense of peace and something that feels like joy. This new peacefulness seems to coincide with the lessons in creativity with watercolors I mentioned earlier. I set aside time to "play" with creativity each day. Not only that, but I convinced my husband it would be fun for us to do this together as well as reaping benefits in ramping up his creativity as he is doing some writing. I convinced him these creative playtimes could be just the thing for writer's block. So we starting sharing what one of the authors of the creativity book called "yoga for the mind." Soon we were looking forward to those sessions of creating something just for fun each day. I am sure that the fact that I was able to get to my second school workshop (no blizzard that day!) and it went well and was very enjoyable contributed to my positive attitude. But this sense of acceptance and calm is more than creativity sessions or work successfully completed. It has gradually unfolded over many days of living in a silent, beautiful cocoon of snow and ice. It continues to grow when I reach out and form relationships with others in our isolated situation. I spent an afternoon with a talented and interesting group of women who shared fascinating stories of their roots in the community (4 generations of women for one) and their various talents of quilt-making, photography and etching intricate pictures of wildlife. My husband and I had a relaxed dinner with neighbors while a storm howled outside. I shared a rich conversation over a two-hour cup of coffee at a local bookstore back in Indiana with a friend whose thoughtful insights stretched my thinking and challenged me. All of these experiences made me aware that if we slow down and pay attention, we can be incredibly enriched by the people around us, those people we formerly have not been in the habit of making time for in our busy working lives. And that simple experiences and quiet days can be incredibly nourishing.

I had a conversation with a woman I recently met whose husband has just retired from the diplomatic corps. They left the busyness of Washington and moved all their belongings to their summer home on Lake Michigan with plans to live there year round. She said that she likes to be bored sometimes because then she is forced to get in touch with herself and decide how she really would like to spend her time instead of having her time controlled from outside. I am starting to understand that.

I don't know how to explain clearly where I am now except to say that I'm happy!

To be clear, I'm not watching daytime TV nor am I taking long naps (well, maybe sometimes.) I'm not "vegging." But I am taking time and I do feel comfortable in my skin—at least right now. I'm enjoying simple things without feeling the rather frantic push to accomplish too much in a short time that has been my mindset for so long. I still give a lot of thought to projects I would be interested in pursuing. I do believe that the time will be right for me to carry out one or more of them, in fact I still have an inner feeling that I am on the cusp of something. The difference now is that I don't feel I need to push or strive to create something so that I can prove myself. It's not the desire that's different, it is the pushing and striving that have shifted. **I want my life to be an unfolding, not a struggle.**

I think I am at the point where I can see this stage of my life as truly a new beginning. Every day is a day of discovery. Before, I believe that I thought of these years as more of a transition to something that I hoped would be good and enjoyable, but that would, in any case, be somewhat inferior to my young adult years, sort of a pallid add-on.

As we go through our lives we look forward to the next stage with great optimism. "When I grow up," "When I can drive," "When I get married," "When I have children" are all milestones that are greeted with enthusiasm. The milestone of retirement evokes very different emotions. Instead of being excited about what this new life stage will bring, we greet it with grim determination to square our shoulders and work with valor to make lemonade out of lemons. We are determined to "put on our big girl pants and start walking" in the words of a phrase I use frequently. But does it have to be like that?

I do feel different. I do not want to live a retread of who I was in my career. It is a new adventure as I discover new facets of myself. On the other hand, I am learning to be cautious about being overconfident that "I have this thing whipped." There have been too many times in my life when I believed I had everything in place only to be dismayed by how little I can actually control. I am also aware that even in the 7 months I have been writing this I have been through an incredible range of ups and downs. I know there are days when I feel on top of the world with my creative juices flowing and then there are other days when I am sunk in gloom, convinced that everything is downhill from here. This transitional time in my life has taught me that change is the only constant, so next month's entry may be quite different. However, I do believe I am growing and learning and I'm looking forward to seeing the magic of hope and change.

8

Is There a Pattern Here?

> "You can't connect the dots looking forward; you can only connect them looking backwards. So you have to trust that the dots will somehow connect in your future."
>
> — Steve Jobs

A PHONE CALL from a sweet, soft-spoken grandmother from New Orleans made me stop and think. She had found my contact information from my special education website and called to ask about establishing an IEP (Individualized Educational Plan) for her 2nd grade grandson. She spoke of him with great pride making sure that I knew that even though he struggles with reading, he is a whiz at math and "the most polite little boy you would ever want to meet." The reason she had called was, as she said, "I have these questions about what to do to help my grandson in school and I don't have anyone to ask." We talked for quite a while and I helped her understand what she needed to do to get an IEP in place and she told me stories about her grandson. At the end of our conversation she said, "Thank you so much for listening to me, Doctor." I sat for a long time afterward holding the phone and thinking.

I am contacted periodically by people who have a child with a disability and who don't know where to turn for advice. The calls come from all over the country. A father from Georgia had no idea what an IEP is, but he had heard that it might help his 6th grade daughter learn to read. A distraught young mother from Spokane, sobbed softly on the phone as she told me that the local public school had agreed to provide speech therapy for her nonverbal preschooler. The problem was that the day care center he attended was refusing to provide someone to wait outside with the little boy for the school bus to arrive and yet the bus couldn't pick him up at the door because it didn't fit under the canopy of the day care building. This mother was seeing her hopes to get help for her child fade because the school and day care were unable to reach a compromise. I share my knowledge and experience with these callers and assist them to the best of my ability. It is truly a service because it certainly is not a "business." I am rarely paid, partly because I don't ask. I am unable to tell that grandmother or any of the other struggling parents and grandparents who call me that I would be happy to answer their questions—for a fee. I do agree with a friend who told me that the wisdom I have gathered through the years is valuable and I should never hesitate to ask for recompense for my knowledge. I believe that people are absolutely correct in charging for valuable services. It's just that I can't do it. My main reason is that I believe that many of my callers would struggle to be able to pay for my services and so I would in effect be turning away people who most need the advice I can offer. The other reason is that I am arguably the world's worst salesperson. I have always contended that if my family were dependent on my financial acumen and salesmanship, we would all have starved long ago. Thank God for my husband who has kept this ship afloat!

Volunteering our services and giving of ourselves to help others is a long and proud tradition in our society. I have dear friends who have incredibly generous spirits and have given to others in amazing and gracious ways. So why would I hesitate to give freely any help I can provide particularly in an area in which I have unique insight built upon years of experience? A friend who has been a treasured sounding board on this journey describes using what we know in service to others as being truly **magnanimous**. I like that word as well as the thought behind it.

    I feel I am returning once more to a fork in the road with no clear idea of how the dots will connect. To add to my confusion, I was talking about this issue with a close friend who knows my love for quotes. She shared, "**The master sticks to (her) tools**" by Lao-Tzu. Hmm. So I am back to asking myself questions and listening for some clarity. On one hand I think that maybe it is better to stick with what I know and can do well rather than striking out in new directions. But, I look forward to making art and love doing it. The main question is about where my art fits in the overall picture. Is creating art really my main avenue to fulfillment or should it be something I love doing that gives my life richness and joy? Is there something more for me to do? Did my art take center stage temporarily to give me time and space to think through what I needed to think through? I know doing art will continue to have a large part in my life. It's the "miracle" that I can point to as the touchstone of my new way of living. It's just a question of whether there are other parts to fit into this puzzle also and how it all fits together.

    I think this whole issue of balancing meaning and enjoyment and how that balance leads to fulfillment is at the crux of what many of us struggle with in this life stage. The years spent in our careers and vocations and our life experiences have given each of us unique and valuable wisdom. Many of us believe, as I do, that what we did with our lives wasn't a random choice, but that there was a clear purpose behind the direction we chose. The question then becomes: was that purpose only for a season or is there value in continuing to live our passion in another form? The axiom that I have lived by is that I want to leave the world a better place because I was here. Have I fulfilled that goal or is there still more to do? As I said earlier, I don't believe we are meant to try to fashion our lives into a retread of our former careers. I don't believe that attempting to re-do what we did before in diminished ways is the path to fulfillment. If there were still a place that would work for us in the institutional structure we formerly inhabited, we would probably not have retired in the first place. The way forward doesn't lie in turning back, so I think whatever we choose to do needs to be fresh and unconventional. It needs to be truly a new beginning and, at least for me, it needs to be done in the spirit of magnanimity and compassion.

I am thinking that this may be the guidance our generation of trail blazing women can give to women following us. Maybe **we** are the ones who can lead the way into discovering creative and unique ways of continuing to contribute without grasping fearfully to what has been. We can be the ones to demonstrate by our lives that the mindset that retirement as an either-or-proposition of either continuing to work in traditional ways or having no involvement at all in our area of expertise is out-of-date and limiting. We need bold thinking that moves away from the way things have always been done. I believe we women are the ones who are most able to do that.

In the meantime I am still finding great joy in painting. In fact I have started a series of nursery rhyme illustrations just for fun. Even though they started as simply a fun project, they have turned into something much more. My children enjoyed the whimsical illustrations so much that they requested that I make a nursery rhyme book for each of the grandchildren. I also continue to spend some time creating art every day and on many days the time in front of my easel is truly the highlight of the day.

Three months into my retirement I wrote that my IEP service was a flawed business plan. I had come to terms with the idea that the way in which I planned to continue doing what had been essentially my life's work was basically untenable. So I moved on, realizing that starting fresh means moving into new and unexplored directions. I still believe in the magic of new beginnings and looking at things with fresh eyes. But, now, five months later, I am rethinking and wondering if there might possibly be value there after all. I know this sounds indecisive and a bit muddled, but certain factors are entering into my thinking. For one thing, even though I have done very little to update my web site or to reach out to customers, people are still calling periodically and their needs and questions are compelling. But the most important change is that I realized the way I had planned on providing my services wasn't workable because it didn't fit for me. It was when I began looking with fresh eyes at what people are searching for and the specific value I add, that I began seeing things differently. Most of the people who have contacted me for advice—parents and educators alike—are simply confused and frustrated and need help in understanding what to do. In addition, I have had an excellent response to several white papers I have written and posted on my website explaining different aspects of special education. This leads me to believe that the best service I can provide is to be available to give information; help clear up confusion; or even, as in the case of the grandmother in New Orleans, just simply listen. I don't have any illusions, for all the reasons I recounted back in November, that I will be inundated with clients. And I have no interest in "scaling" a business or scrambling to try to figure out the necessary complex technology to be successful. (I found early on that path only leads to teeth-grinding frustration for me.) But I think there is value in being there for the people, even if only a few, who really need help. So, now I need to reflect on how that would look and wait to see if "the way to do it becomes clear."

There is another dot I hope will be connected and that has to do with reaching out and joining with other women in making this journey of transition. I have found great strength in the conversations I have had around this subject with my wise and strong women friends. I have been amazed at how many women say "me too" when I share my story or admit that they are worried about a friend who is struggling with this same transition. My husband was at a meeting recently and some issues surrounding retirement came up. One of the participants, an extremely articulate woman in a leadership position, turned to my husband and told him that she is retiring in 3 months and she is "scared to death." This is a smart, competent woman with a supportive, close family and many interests. I think that what she fears is what she believes she will be losing in the transition. I think most of us have a feeling of loss, but more than that, I think we feel a sort of existential loneliness. That feeling isn't an "aloneness," because many of us have close families who are precious to us, and many special people around us. I think it is more of a need to connect with others who are at our same point in life and who understand what we are feeling or, maybe even more, a need to learn from women who are ahead of us on this path and can help point the way. I have heard it said that one of women's strengths is that we are able to be open and vulnerable. I believe this is true, but only if we carve out the time and create vehicles to encourage each other. The importance of supporting and learning from each other as we move forward cannot be overemphasized in my mind and—even better—it makes the journey so much more fun!

9

"Guts and Honor"

"And the day came when the risk to remain tight in a bud was more painful than the risk it took to blossom."

— Anais Nin

IT WAS ONE of those stories on NPR that made me sit in my car in the garage unable to shut off the engine until the end. Returning home from a Saturday afternoon of running errands, I was casually listening to a humorous report about a quirky new fad in San Francisco (of course.) Apparently the latest "foodie" trend is—toast. Yes, that comfort food breakfast staple and faithful standby of busy parents everywhere has been elevated to gourmet status in certain trendy restaurants. I was enjoying listening and trying to puzzle out why so many people are paying big bucks for a humble piece of toast when the story shifted. The focus turned to a young woman who owns an eccentric little restaurant in a far-from-fashionable neighborhood in San Francisco. It was an amazing story about 34 year old Guiletta Carrelli and her restaurant with the improbable name of **The Trouble Coffee and Coconut Club.** She only serves three menu items: toast, coconuts and freshly-squeezed grapefruit juice and her unique approach to her life is illustrated by the fact that she calls the drip coffee at her restaurant "guts" while the espresso is called "honor."

Google the restaurant. You will be captivated by this heartwarming tale. I don't want to ruin it for you, you need to read it for yourself, but there were several profound thoughts that I can't get out of my head.

One of the points made in the article is that most of us spend the majority of our time with significant others such as family and very close friends. However, Ms. Carelli has struggled throughout her life with mental health issues and it became clear to her that those kinds of close primary ties would become overwhelmed by her needs if they were all she had to depend on. So that's where her restaurant comes in. The restaurant has become her community. She has developed relationships and forged ties with both the regulars at her restaurant and friends in the neighborhood. I certainly am not suggesting that any of us has mental health issues or that we should go out and start a restaurant. I value tremendously those special, irreplaceable ties with my loved ones. But I do think that if we depend on our families and those few other extremely close relationships to be our sole support system and the source of our happiness, we may be expecting a lot and setting ourselves up for some problems including my biggest fear—becoming a "burden." Many of us have been too busy for most of our lives to form those kinds of ties. Working, raising a family and trying to be good daughters ourselves has left us very little time through the years for casual friendships. In addition, although hopefully women today are mentally healthier in this regard, guilt played a large part in how I chose to spend my time. The time I spent away from my children working needed to be made up by spending extra "quality time." This elusive use of extra hours that made me feel better about myself could be anything from being assistant cub leader for my son's troop to serving as team mother for my daughter's volleyball team. Anything to avoid the self-punishing fear of being selfish or, even worse, being a neglectful mother. Now that time seems to be speeding up, we think a lot about it—how to spend it, how little there is of it, how did it manage to speed by so quickly? I think we can all agree that there are a lot of positives to having more of it.

Developing new friendships may be one of them. This may be one of the benefits of this thing called retirement. It may even offset for me the down side of having more leisure time on my hands than I think I would like to have. Despite my somewhat ambivalent feelings about time, I do know I would rather go out and participate and meet new people than validate today's LA Times crossword puzzle definition for "retired." (Yes, I admit I enjoy doing crossword puzzles every once in awhile. After all, how else could I find out such valuable information as the name of the last Oldsmobile model ever made?) As I filled in the blanks for the answer of their idea of retirement, I found to my amazement and wrath the answer was "put out to pasture." How sensitive of the LA Times!

The second profound and important moment for me in Ms. Carrelli's story was a question that her older friend and mentor asked Ms. Carrelli when she was still struggling to figure things out during the time before she started her restaurant. He asked her, "**What is your useful skill in a tangible situation?**" What an insightful question! Rather than dreaming about what we might do "if only..." this pushes us in the direction of practical, grounded reality. It forces us to get honest with ourselves. Determining in our minds the answer to this question can point a beacon to what our lives should look like and the direction for our next steps. It is a cop-out when we say that we are planning on doing something we know very well isn't really a realistic option and yet it gives us an excuse when it inevitably fails.

I love the well-known question, "**What would you do if you weren't afraid to fail?**" I think it is a fascinating and important thing to think about. The problem is, I am not sure many of us can answer for sure because, at least for me, it is so hypothetical. I have lived my whole life with a fear of failure and therefore I am not sure I would be able to recognize what it would feel like to not have that fear. However, assessing what our strengths have been in practical situations forces us to take stock of who we really are and what we actually can do. I believe we all have very tangible and tested real strengths and valuable gifts.

I spent three days in the hospital last week. Lying in a hospital room provides plenty of time to think. In the middle of the night on an impossibly skinny bed covered with plastic that crackled every time I turned, there wasn't much else to do. Sleep is certainly not a realistic option. This hospital stay was not the result of another disaster like I experienced last December. This stay was due to a pretty common piece of the aging process, atrial fibrillation, that my cardiologist hoped would be addressed in my case by a new medication. The clue to the commonality of this condition is the increasing number of advertisements aimed at our demographic showing attractive and healthy older adults going about their daily lives with everything controlled by the advertised miracle drug. I have had atrial fibrillation (uneven heart beat) for four years and have been on blood thinners, beta blockers and other medications that control it, but don't "fix" it. My cardiologist is determined to "fix" it. So I was in the hospital while they monitored my reaction to the new medication. If all went well, at the end of these days of forced, mind-numbing idleness, they would "zap" my heart and it would be shocked into normalcy or, as one of my nurses put it, "the normal rhythm that's inside will be let out." When I asked what would happen if there was no normal rhythm inside clamoring to be set free, the answer was a smile and a shrug.

In the dim glow from the corridor I thought about all the people lying in the darkness like me alone with their thoughts while their monitors beeped. In an effort to combat total, mind-numbing boredom, I had walked the halls that afternoon and as I peeked into the rooms in passing I saw that most of the occupants are elderly and many of them seem pretty sick. It is a heart hospital so that would be expected. I thought of all the accumulated life stories in those rooms and I felt pretty sure that very few of these people ever thought they would be in this place when they were young and just starting out on their lives. They certainly would never have chosen this and if there was a way they could have avoided being here in this place I have little doubt they would have taken it. It came to me that the aging process is one of the only things in life I have encountered that I cannot overcome by sheer grit and determination. There is no stopping it, no work-around, no alternative path. It's never easy to be part of an end of an era, even if it is someone else's "decline." Golf analyst Jay Busbee in an article on-line at the time of the recent Master's golf tournament when neither Tiger Woods nor Phil Mickelson made the finals noted that they both are on the **"downslope of their careers and there's sadness in that, both because it's happened and because we've got a lot more of that kind of thing ahead."** As Busbee gloomily reminds us, the inevitable side effects of aging will become more common and even familiar. But so will the good things like the fun I had this evening "Face Timing" with my grandchildren, Ana and Nate, to wish me luck on my "heart zapping" and so that Ana could shut the door to her bedroom and share a special secret about her day with me, face-to-face from 200 miles away!

The "zapping" procedure (technically called cardio-version) didn't work. The cardiologist said that my heart beat a grand total of 3 times in perfect rhythm and then reverted to its jaggedly uneven self. Although I am willing to accept the fact that seemingly there is no regular beat imprisoned within my heart, my doctors are determined to try again in 10 days. I will come in as an outpatient and, hopefully, will leave with a perfect heart rhythm. I think I am more philosophical and accepting of my imperfect heartbeat than the doctors are. One of the important lessons I have begun to learn on this year's journey is that some things cannot be controlled. Some things just "are" no matter how much we wish they could be different. I am feeling that I am, at least a bit, more in tune with the inevitable ebb and flow of life with its ups and downs, frustrations, and strange anomalies. I still certainly have my moments, but I feel that I am in a more peaceful place and have less of a need to kick the walls when things don't go the way I think they should.

10

Walking Through New Doors

"When one door of happiness closes, another opens; but often we look so long at the closed door that we do not see the one which has opened for us."

— Helen Keller

WHEN I READ Helen Keller's words in this quote, I wonder why they are true. Why is it so hard for so many of us to accept new opportunities that are available to us? Why do we remain mired in regret? The most obvious reason is that we continue to strongly want what we had so much that we are not open to other possibilities. Our lives are no longer centered around living that particular passion and yet we are still attached to the life we had. But I am not sure the answer is always that simple. That there may be more to this seeming inability to move on came to me as a result of a special hospital visit and a very insightful magazine article. First, the visit.

On one of those days when I was a guest of the hospital (yes, they now call us "guests" as a clever way to make us feel better about why we are there,) I was briskly circling the corridors to get a bit of exercise. As I rounded a corner I came face-to-face with one of my former students and his mother. They had come to visit me. This student has been a very special part of my life. He was already attending Midwest

Academy when I began my tenure as Head of School and he was with me the whole seven years. His graduation and my retirement were on the same day and, in fact, he and I walked out of the ceremony arm-in-arm leading the graduation recessional. He is the bravest and kindest young men I have ever met and it is a privilege to know him and his equally special family. He has Asperger's syndrome, but in addition, he contracted leukemia when he was in high school. Neither of those conditions broke his spirit. Even though he has had many months of chemotherapy treatments and has spent a large portion of his teen-age years in the hospital, he remains unfailingly polite and cheerful. I remember his smiling face hanging from the car window when his mother brought him to school to visit. Because of his almost non-existent immune system at the height of the leukemia, he could not be in range of all those "kid germs" so his mother and I made arrangements that she would pull into the parking lot at school and we would bring the students out to stand around the car and talk with him. On the evening when we both graduated I called him up to the stage before the recessional and he and I, arm-in-arm, led the other graduates from the hall. Although he was leaning heavily on his cane, and he was clearly in pain, his proud smile warmed everyone's heart. He is doing well. He has only 2 more chemotherapy treatments to go and I am so happy for him. I have remained friends with his mother also and she had been texting me funny messages while I was in the hospital to lift my spirits. One of the reasons they came to the hospital was that they had visited the Chihuly glass museum while on a family trip and knowing that I love blown glass, he took pictures of the exhibits on his cell phone and thought bringing them to show me would be just the ticket to cheer me up. It was. This young man is extremely sensitive and attuned to other's feelings (proving that stereotypes of young people with Asperger's syndrome are just that—stereotypes.) As we talked in my hospital room he made an extremely perceptive comment. He said, "You know Dr. Stoughton in your last months at Midwest, I could tell that you were getting tired." He thought a minute and then amended his statement to, "Well, maybe not tired but...you seemed like you were looking for something new, like a new challenge." Pretty sharp I would say. It was true. My journal entries said it, my family and friends knew it, and yet I have had difficulty walking away from the closed door and finding the new doors to happiness that are open. Why? That is where the magazine article comes in.

After I came home from the hospital, I picked up an issue of *Atlantic Monthly* and began reading—actually devouring—an article by two women journalists, Katty Kay and Claire Shipman, titled "The Confidence Gap." I believe that anyone who knows me would attest to the fact that I am generally a confident woman. Many experiences that others find traumatic like speaking in front of people, standing up for what I believe, and truly thinking that I can do anything I set my mind to are a piece of cake (Actually in the spirit of full disclosure roller coasters and other thrill rides make me quake in fear, but I'm pretty much able to avoid those things.) However, according to Kay and Shipman, even women who are at the high end of the confidence scale can have certain issues that bar them from being truly self-assured. There are two prominent areas that women struggle with. First, is our difficulty to step out boldly in areas that we perceive carry a risk of failure. This causes us to obsess about our performance and strive for perfection. As children, to a greater or lesser extent depending on our other personality traits, we learn that being a "good girl" is rewarded. We find that there is great value in doing things the "right way." I laughed when I read the words of Stanford psychology professor, Carol Dweck, who was quoted in the article as saying that, "**If life were one long grade school, women would be the undisputed leaders of the world."** I laughed because I remembered my grade school self sitting in the front row waving my hand in the air incessantly to answer any and all questions. Sheryl Sandberg's campaign against calling girls "bossy" was tailor-made for me. I also laughed because every time during my life when I needed to feel good about myself, I would attend classes. It did the trick. I would accumulate some A's and plenty of positive feedback and suddenly all was right with the world again. It is such a marked pattern for me that recently when I was having some down feelings about my life, my husband helpfully—and very seriously—suggested that I might want to go back to school! I have four advanced degrees because, to paraphrase the common saying, when the going gets tough, I go back to school.

The second issue that is a common problem for women is our hesitancy to advocate for ourselves. A solid body of research shows that women ask for salary increases less frequently than men and when we do ask, we tend to ask for much more modest amounts. We generally are poor negotiators for ourselves in every area. This is a real problem for me. I have never actually negotiated a salary increase. Instead I have relied on a boss or a board to take the lead in rewarding me for my hard work. I, of course, received raises, bonuses and promotions during my working years, but they were a natural consequence of the system of which I was a part or a reward bestowed on me for work well done rather than being initiated by me. When I retired, one of my biggest regrets is that I had no idea how to negotiate my exit. I had no experience with that sort of thing, nor any mentor to guide me in how to do it. I had fleeting thoughts of hiring someone to guide me through the process, but I didn't know even where to turn to find the right person. I firmly believe this whole area of self-advocacy is an important issue for many more women than we realize.

It is easy to see why an article on confidence is important to take to heart if you are still in the working world and in the midst of trying to climb the corporate ladder. But what does this discussion have to do with those of us who are at a very different place in our lives? Further, what is the connection with Helen Keller's doors? I believe that, somewhat counter-intuitively, we need self-assurance at this stage of our lives almost more than at any other time. We aren't functioning within a set structure that tells us what we must do to succeed and advance. There is no external template or set of benchmarks that let us know when we are making it. We are on our own in creating meaning and goals. We only have two choices as Helen Keller points out: we can stare mournfully at closed doors reminiscing about times past and reliving the "glory days, or we can walk through new doors and start creating new memories. We can either dwell in the world of nostalgia or build new experiences. I am totally of the belief that those experiences can be as big and brassy or as simple and quiet as I want them to be. Sometimes I beat myself up because I'm no longer involved in something that is important enough to change the world. But, as I am coming to understand, that kind of thinking is not freedom but rather the ugly head of perfectionism rearing itself up again. What I really want is to feel comfortable enough with who I am that I can ignore that negative, niggling voice in my head that says, "That's a dumb idea," or "You can't do that because you're too (old, unqualified, overqualified, out-of-shape, or out-of-the-loop.") That is where confidence—or lack thereof—comes in. I want the only qualification for what I do to be that when I come to the end of the day I will count it a day well spent and I will feel alive and eager to begin the next day. I want to live without worrying about critical judgments—particularly my own.

Being evaluated is truly painful for me. I remember when I was teaching I would beg the principal to not tell me ahead of time when he planned to visit my classroom for my annual evaluation. An off-the-cuff surprise visit would be fine with me. I knew I was a good teacher, so I had nothing to worry about. Although most teachers would far prefer knowing ahead so they could make sure they had planned a top-flight lesson, I worried, lost sleep and became awash with anxiety because I reasoned that if I knew about the observation ahead of time I would be expected to have planned my very best lesson. The negative little voice whispering in my ear would imagine the principal saying, "And that's your **best?**" The pressure of feeling that my best would be found lacking was miserable.

The option to step out and risk takes a certain level of confidence as a precursor of action. The article said that "**confidence**

is the factor that turns thoughts into judgments about what we are capable of and then transforms those thoughts into action." Action. Hmm. Does that mean taking out the framed pastels I have stacked, still wrapped in brown paper, in my closet risking embarrassment and rejection to actually find out if they are sellable? Does that mean that the reams of pages of writing I have done might serve a better purpose than sitting in colored file folders in a drawer I rarely open? Could it mean that all the knowledge and experience I have gained in my years of teaching might be of benefit to others if I offered it without fear of rejection? Could it be that I have more issues than a fear of roller coasters? I do believe that there is great value in painting a landscape or putting my thoughts down on paper simply because it brings me joy. I just want to make sure that my decisions are a real choice and not based on fear or insecurity. I don't want to limit my horizons because I avoid evaluation. **I wonder if the issue is actually not that I am so attached to the closed door but that I am fearful of giving the open door a try. Could that be the issue with many of us who hold back from what could be exciting opportunities?**

We each have our own issues. Mine is that I am supremely confident and enthusiastic in beginning projects and pursuing ideas, but that enthusiasm isn't always sustained. I have so many ideas and I launch so many new things and yet they often wither due to inaction. This may be why, as kind and encouraging as he is, my husband's eyes glaze over when I start talking about the latest great new idea I have. Right now I have several unfinished writing projects. I have enough pastels finished for a small gallery; I have whimsical water color illustrations for just about every familiar nursery rhyme; and I still, at least in theory, have my special education counseling service. My daughters love the illustrations and want to help me make them into a book even if for no other reason than for their own children to enjoy; my husband is willing to work with me to try to market my pastels; marketing experts have suggested a number of creative ways to broaden my consulting service to reach more people; and there are a number of avenues through which to share my written thoughts with others. I agree with everyone and I make action plans, but then I over-think and back away. I become convinced that what I've done isn't original enough, valuable enough, or good enough. I have completed a 50-page booklet explaining the IEP process in layman's terms. I wrote it to help people who are struggling to obtain the best educational opportunities for their children and don't know what to do. Yet, I have let myself off the hook of doing anything further with it by telling myself that everything I wrote has already been said. As the *Atlantic Monthly* article said, when women hesitate because we aren't sure, we hold ourselves back. I'm not saying that everything I do has to "turn into something" or be an end product. Some things are just fun to do. But I do know, that at least for me, there is a sense of satisfaction and accomplishment in being able to point to a finished product that I worked hard on and feel good about. I would like to know if I just haven't found the right thing yet, or if I just can't seem to complete a project. I also want to be free of the shadow side of the little girl who wanted to answer all the questions. The "bossy" side was only part of my school performance. The other aspect of my intense personality was that I would burst into inconsolable tears whenever I missed a word on a spelling test. I would much rather be "bossy."

The hopeful thing is that it is never too late to build confidence—even later in life. Science tells us that our brains never lose their plasticity or the ability to change and develop. It is never too late to take a risk; fail; get past the embarrassment; and start over again. You realize the world didn't end and you are a bit tougher and wiser. This is where the importance of having a sense of humor and a certain lightness about life and our place in it plays an important part. For example, I have always loved this humorous comment from Eleanor Roosevelt, who in her no-nonsense way says, **"You wouldn't worry so much about what others think of you if you realized how seldom they do."** Although Eleanor Roosevelt is not generally thought of as funny, I chuckle about the way this comment puts things in perspective. I'm no fonder than anyone else of looking foolish or wrong or misguided, but even those unpleasant moments sound better to me than never again having the thrill of anticipation that comes from stepping up and trying something bold and new—and making it happen. The risk of making a mess of things has to be better than living in the past tense. Confidence not only leads to action—it leads to hope.

Oprah turned 60 recently and, coincidentally, she took that opportunity to talk about these very things that are on my mind. She had this to say about passing the milestone of her 60th birthday:

The best part is being free and doing whatever you want. The hardest part is recognizing the time that you've wasted and the things that you worried about that didn't really matter.

Those are good words, and I want to be in that place! However, I suppose that even if you are Oprah, learning to free yourself from trivial worries and having the freedom and strength to do anything you want is not easy. Being high-minded about the things we feel inadequate about does not come easily even in our 60s. I never get over my shock of looking in the mirror and wondering who that older woman is and where those wrinkles came from. I still am as prone to worrying about things I can't change as I ever have been. I still want to be involved in exciting things, but I worry that my time of vital involvement is in the past. I worry about my husband having to bear the full burden of supporting us financially instead of the partnership we have always had. I've got a long way to go before I feel fully free to do whatever I want and I suspect I am not alone. But when I get discouraged, I remember back to the story of my friend and the group of women I talked about earlier. They were there for each other in a rough time in each of their lives and yet they didn't let anyone cling to the safety net of the group. Each woman was encouraged to find a new passion and when that happened, to go follow it. I need that support—friends who will be by my side but who will also tell me to "pull up my big girl pants and start walking" when I get stuck.

Going through this journey has convinced me that we women need each other's encouragement and support and yet we can be so involved in caretaking and helping out and serving others—the things that we women have always done to keep our worlds going—that we can become isolated and lonely. We can risk losing our dreams, or possibly never discovering them. I believe that every woman has something special that she would like to do or be. It may be well hidden, but it's there. I also believe that sometimes it takes some pulling out and encouragement to bring those dreams to the surface. **Too often we convince ourselves that our hopes and dreams are unimportant and unworthy and so we miss out on a beautiful part of life.**

My mother was a quiet, unassuming, very private woman who rarely, if ever talked about herself. I remember her cleaning the house and cooking meals, but I knew little about her inner thoughts. Several years after she died, on a visit to her sister, my 95-year old aunt, I found an exquisitely knitted sweater in palest pink with beautiful pink shell buttons in a drawer carefully wrapped in tissue paper. It was an intricate design and it was perfectly executed. When I asked about this puzzling find my aunt told me that my mother loved to knit and was an expert knitter. I vaguely remember her knitting occasionally when I was little, but I got the impression that it was "no big deal"—just something to keep her hands busy. I certainly would never have known that it was a real joy for her. The fact that I was totally unaware of this talent because she never talked about it leaves me feeling empty and regretful and sad. It also makes me wonder what other hopes and dreams she had that I never knew about. How many of us women never step out and claim a talent or ability or interest that could enrich our lives so deeply—and maybe our daughters' lives as well?

Every time I talk about my late-in-life painting discovery, inevitably someone will say, "You know I always wanted to (you can fill in the blanks), but I never pursued it." The reasons are varied and a little sad, "I was always too busy," "It didn't seem important enough," "I knew it was a silly idea," "I didn't have the talent for it." Right after discovering pastel painting I shared with my staff at a faculty meeting about my new found interest and challenged them to take some time to discover something that would ignite their interest and spark up their lives. Something just for them. One of the teachers responded quietly that she had always wanted to play the piano however, now that she was middle aged she figured it was probably too late. But she took my challenge to heart and signed up for piano lessons and she is happily playing the piano today.

Because I believe in women helping women, I have decided to take an action step and I am actually following through with it. I have invited a small group of like-minded women to come together and talk about how we can support each other. We are meeting next week and I am excited to see what this conversation will bring. Women I share my story with tell me that I am expressing exactly where they are and they say how relieved they are to know they are not alone in those feelings. We can share expertise as well as emotional support. We can help each other find our way. I can't wait to see where the path leads.

11

Claiming my Inner Strength

> "Twenty years from now you will be more disappointed by the things you didn't do than by the things you did do. So throw off the bowlines. Sail away from the safe harbor. Catch the trade winds in your sails. Explore. Dream. Discover."
>
> — Mark Twain

ONE OF THE things that people who retire are "supposed to do" is travel. I have always loved traveling. I visited Europe 5 times by the age of 19 because my father was a college professor who used his sabbaticals to see the world. Many of my children's favorite memories are centered around family vacations. I also agree that this time of life with our lessened responsibilities and more flexible schedules is a good time to visit places we have long wanted to see and learn about. So when long-time friends invited us to join them for a week at a timeshare in Tuscany, I jumped at the chance. Here was yet another experience to add to this year of experiences. I felt this was an important move to shake up a routine that has become a bit too predictable, comfortable and safe. It became even clearer how much I needed to do this because, as the time for departure drew closer, I felt a mix of eager anticipation and hesitancy to leave my comfort zone. The truth is that foreign travel is both great fun and a hassle and dragging around paraphernalia like sleep machines and dealing with a heart that has its own idiosyncratic rhythm is a far cry from my 20-year old carefree days of backpack traveling including spending the night in a Volkswagon bug in the middle of the Libyan dessert. But I was looking forward to this trip very much and I was quite sure that once I broke out of my routine I would have a great time.

It didn't seem to make much sense to limit ourselves to only one week in Italy, so I planned travels for my husband and me in Switzerland for the week preceding meeting our friends in Italy. I looked at this experience as another piece in this yearlong research process. It would help us decide if travel is enough, or even almost enough, as a purpose for the upcoming years. Our friends who have retired are pretty evenly divided between those who partition their year between a couple of permanent or semi-permanent residences in different locations and those who take frequent trips instead of relocating. So far in these pages I have chronicled our adventures in our choice of the first alternative—living for a good part of the year in Michigan—and we are pretty solid on the pros and cons of that. Now the opportunity is available to check out the travel option. What we do know is that we are not interested in the choice that many older travelers are taking to leave the planning to others through tours or cruises or riverboat trips. We are in agreement that we want to be in charge of our activities and our time. We want to be able to wander the streets people-watching at our leisure rather than having to follow an imposed schedule. There is also a certain amount of self-testing involved. Can we navigate independent travel and deal with hotels, trains, planes, and language differences using only our own resources or is that too difficult at this stage in our lives? Since one theme for me this year has been to challenge myself and to focus on living forward without being tangled in self-imposed barriers, how this turns out is important. My goal for myself and those of you who are sharing my journey through these pages is not to get off track with a "My Trip to Europe" travelogue. (Don't worry, I will also spare you the 367 photographs I took.) I want to be true to my purpose and simply share what I learned about myself and how this new set of experiences impacts the life I want to live. So I stuck a blank journal in my suitcase to record any thoughts and revelations and set off on the plane on a cool evening in early May heading for our first stop in Zurich—and adventure.

Two learning experiences stand out as significant. One has to do with overcoming self-imposed barriers and the other is about living life fully and with open arms.

Walking the Ramparts.
Stepping out of my comfort zone; overcoming barriers that make me feel safe and yet that make my life less full; and thinking deeply about the meaning of passion and its place in my life seem to be the main lessons my trip to Europe presented to me.

First the difficulty with barriers. This lesson can be expressed in three words: "Walking the Ramparts." In both Lucerne and a lovely little walled town we visited on a "train field trip" through the Swiss Alps from Bern, there were opportunities to walk along the top of the ancient town wall. The tops of the walls, or ramparts, in these ancient walled cities provided a panoramic view of the surrounding countryside to the soldiers who were guarding the town in medieval times. Although parts of them have crumbled with age, the sections of wall that remain provide the same gorgeous view for people who walk along them today. My first wall-walking opportunity was in Lucerne. I **really** wanted to walk those ramparts so I set off for the wall, camera in hand, preparing to take breathtaking photos that I would later turn into landscape paintings. In hunting for the obscure way to enter the wall we finally discovered that getting to the ramparts involved entering a cramped, dark guardhouse and climbing narrow steep wooden steps—seemingly hundreds of them—that ascended straight up. I stood at the bottom looking up—way, way up—to where I could see a distant patch of blue sky. It hit me that I should have realized how high the walls were as their purpose was protection. What good would a little dinky wall have done? But at any rate, there was everything wrong with this picture for me personally including the steepness of the stairs, their claustrophobic closeness and darkness, and the realization that I would have to come back down after my walk which triggered flashbacks of my traumatic fall down stairs much less vertical than these. I also have been struggling a bit with shortness of breath in connection with my atrial fibrillation and it is most pronounced when climbing stairs. I have to admit honestly that although I have a pretty high threshold for pain and am not inordinately "wimpy" about my health and well-being, the current uncertainty about what is going on with my heart makes me more nervous than usual. So my head became filled with a composite vision of finding myself out of breath and dizzy halfway through a skinny, dark flight of rickety stairs. I made my decision, handed the camera to my husband, and sat down on a bench to wait for him to return telling myself that it was no big deal to miss this one thing. After all, there were so many beautiful things to see in the town and what's one more lovely view. I continued to sit, enjoying the sun on my face and the smell of flowering trees in this peaceful spot while convincing myself that I was perfectly happy with my choice to not take the rampart stroll. But then that pesky voice in my head started talking, telling me that I have never been a fearful person. That voice also reminded me of my determination to continue to be a "take life by the horns" woman not allowing myself to fall into the cautious, timid mode that can creep up on us so easily as we become older. I became increasingly uncomfortable about missing an experience I had looked forward to because of my worries. It felt limiting and sad. I remembered the words of Georgia O'Keefe that, **"I've been absolutely terrified every moment of my life and I've never let it keep me from doing what I wanted to do."**

So, I reversed my decision. I stood up, set my jaw and forced myself to march up those stairs. As I walked along the rampart, I felt strong and happy. The view was remarkable and it was a beautiful day. I certainly took enough photos to fill an art gallery with "pastel landscapes by Edy," but more important, I had not allowed myself to be stopped for the wrong reasons from something I really wanted to do. Climbing to the top of a city wall isn't earth shaking. I didn't decide to go bungee jumping or join a mountain climbing expedition. But it is often in an accumulation of little ways that we almost unconsciously can become passive passengers in our own lives. Drip-by-drip the slow attrition of our confidence turns us into people who turn away rather than embracing the things that are hard for us. Sometimes I think we set ourselves up to fail by focusing on ambitious, unattainable goals. When we don't reach them we convince ourselves that we were right in the first place, we really couldn't do it. If we work on real, practical changes, stretching ourselves in more mundane moments in ways that we can be successful, we have a chance for real, meaningful change. One hill (notice I didn't say mountain) climbed leads us to have the confidence to tackle the next one.

Rachel Simmons, co-founder of Girls' Leadership Institute put this whole idea much better than I can when she wrote about the well-known advice to do one thing that scares you every day. Her response is, "**Who wants to be scared every day? How about do one thing every day that makes you slightly nervous? Not as catchy I know, but that's actually the way real meaningful change happens.**" I think she is absolutely right and that's the way it was with the ramparts. I wasn't frightened, I was slightly nervous. I can deal with, and move past, nervousness. I had the rather humbling experience the other day of reading through some of my old journals. I saw them in a pile on top of a bookcase and decided to sort through them. It was darkly funny to read—back as far as 1990—the hugely ambitious plans I had carved out and the giant steps I planned to take. The humorous part is how similar they were. Each year I would commit myself to pretty much the same grandiose endeavors only to re-commit the next year when I never got there. I think we all need a goal. I know I do. But sometimes it is best to break that overriding, top-of-the-mountain goal into manageable steps. Someone once wisely told me, **"Perfect is the enemy of done."** I think it's important for me to get some small steps under my belt rather than feeling anxious and guilty about my failure to scale the heights.

As I have confessed before in these pages, one of the unfortunate consequences for me in this whole retirement period is that in some ways I feel less confident and bold. I realized that there were limits to my life plans and I began doubting myself more and stepping back from challenges rather than my typical response of jumping in. I have become more introspective and less ready to rush into something too quickly. Both of these are good things. But when they come with attitudes of "That's an exciting idea but"... ("I'm too old," "It's too much trouble," or "I don't have the energy for that kind of thing anymore") they can get in our way. I don't miss the impulsiveness that has dogged my steps through the years, but on the other hand I don't want to lose the enthusiasm and the passion. On those ramparts I feel that in some small way I took a step toward reclaiming myself and my personal strength. It felt good. What would you do if you weren't afraid? What are the ramparts in your life?

Find what you love and do it.
There's a lot of "fake" passion going around in today's society. It appears that becoming a buzzword doesn't do a lot to enhance a concept. On a daily basis we hear, "I'm so passionate about_____" or "_____is my passion" (you can fill in the blanks) and we often get the feeling that there isn't much depth of feeling there. The other day someone on television told me he was "passionate" about selling me a car. It's really too bad because true passion is such an important part of life. A life without passion (the real thing) is dull and lifeless. I don't think that what you are passionate about has to change the world nor does it need to be earthshaking or dramatic. It can be important just to you. But in order to qualify as a passion it is my belief that it should be something that gives us joy and is deeply meaningful to us. It should add zest to our lives and give us a reason to get up in the morning.

One of the great things about passion is that it is infectious. I recently read a statement that sums it up in such a nice way. I am unable to find the name of the person who said it, but I appreciate the wise words. It went like this:

When we focus on leading a passionate, meaningful life, we are also inadvertently creating a spectacular ripple effect of inspiration in the lives around us. When one person follows a dream, tries something new, or takes a daring leap, everyone nearby feels their passionate energy; and before too long, they are making their own daring leaps while simultaneously inspiring others.

What a beautiful way of describing what we women can do for each other if we form a supportive coalition and help each other.

There is definitely real passion out there. One afternoon in Tuscany I had the privilege of encountering authentic passion in an unexpected way. It changed and enriched my life.

The timeshare that our friends had found is brand new. In fact we were among the first people to stay there and the lack of signage meant that what should have been a half hour drive from Pisa ended up taking about 3 hours of winding back and forth on twisting and narrow country roads that we shared with Italian drivers who all seemed to believe they were participating in a road race. The drive was certainly worth it as we found ourselves tucked away in a remote part of Tuscany amidst beautiful vineyards and improbably green rolling hills each topped by a castle rising above ancient walls and parapets. It was profoundly gorgeous. The sleepy little neighboring hilltop town of Pecciolli had a small tourist bureau run by a personable and energetic young man named Massimo. Massimo had the vision that the people who would soon start coming to stay at the timeshare might be interested in some local experiences. This would be a benefit to both the tourists and the local economy. In addition to arranging walking tours of the town, he developed cooking classes to be held in a local agri-tourisma farmhouse. There were several options including making pizza in a huge outdoor stone oven. We signed up for an afternoon of cooking a 4-course Tuscan dinner. I wasn't sure what to expect. I hoped it would be low-key and natural rather than a production staged for tourists. I needn't have worried. The four of us, joined by 3 women from the British Isles, followed our guide Massimo down a long tree-lined country driveway to a lovely little farmhouse where a huge timbre-ceilinged kitchen—and Carla—were waiting for us. Carla was the cook. She was funny, expressive, quick and sure in her actions. In short, she was quintessentially Italian. She was clearly someone who knew what she was doing and was in control of the kitchen She also didn't speak English. So Massimo remained with us the whole time as our translator. It was an amazing experience. We made pasta by hand and diced vegetables with an intimidating-looking tool that looked frighteningly like a scimitar and was called a mezzaluna. We chopped strawberries and dipped special cookies in the juice to make strawberry tiramasu. (In the spirit of full disclosure I almost single-handedly ruined the tiramasu because we needed to whip egg whites and I—with my misguided confidence—offered to crack the eggs. With a flourish as everyone watched I dumped the yolk accidentally into the egg white greatly increasing the difficulty of ever being able to get it beaten properly.) My clumsiness clearly tried Carla's soul but, like all the Italians we met she was very gracious about it (although I have to admit I wasn't sure what she was saying in Italian.)

The end result was a mouth-watering meal that we ate on a picnic table in the yard in the soft mellow colors of a country sunset.

Carla's love for cooking and her skill in the kitchen were indeed inspiring. There was definitely passion there in preparing a beautiful meal. But the truly inspirational part for me was when Massimo talked about food. He was what can only be described simply as someone who deeply respects and loves food. He had carefully selected all the ingredients by hand from local markets and farms to make sure that we were working with only the freshest and best ingredients. But it was when he actually talked about the food and the food preparation that his passion became irresistible. The history of Italian food (including the farms and people who produce it), the importance of selecting only the best ingredients and how to know what the best is, and the respectful and thoughtful way he talked about preparing the food were all part of what he shared with us. His face lit up when he talked about how to cook properly and he clearly was passionate about doing it right. It was more a ritual of good living, hospitality and creativity than a process of simply putting food on the table. He shared an abundance of knowledge in his detailed explanation of the characteristics and importance of extra virgin olive oil, for example, and it was fascinating. I will never look at olive oil the same way again and I promise I will not allow myself to be even in the same room with a food processor. I was inspired by the clear joy that Massimo took in good food cooked well and the art and love that goes into preparing it. I can get in that joyful place when I am creating art, or even sometimes in simply talking about art, so I have known that particular pleasure. My wish for all of us is that we find that. Someone said to me once years ago that there are three things that everyone should try to do before they die: plant a tree, write a book and love a child. Anything from lovingly preparing a meal, to creating pottery, to tending a garden, to taking a class, to reading a story to a child is fair game. It's different for each of us. It can't be just busyness. A friend who lives in an over 55-community told me recently that the women who live there joke that they are "so busy they need to un-retire to relax." But I wonder about that busyness. I hope they are all doing something they love rather than what an acquaintance recently said about her life in retirement, "Well, you just fill your time and hope to enjoy the day." There are many things we can fill our time with and many of them are enjoyable. But, for me at least, there has to be more than filling time. It has to be something I really care about. I have a friend who every year creates a flower garden so beautiful that the colors and aromas make you want to sit in it with a good book and never leave. I, on the other hand, have never met a plant I don't destroy. I like to cook, but could never be as deeply absorbed in it as Massimo is. So there is something different for everyone. But there **is** something for each of us—something that brings a smile to our face.

I have a favorite coffee that I always buy from our local grocery store in Michigan. Larry's Coffee isn't just good coffee. They do everything a coffee company should do. Their coffee is shade grown on family farms with careful environmental responsibility. Each bag of their coffee contains the following words: **"We think life is richer & more rewarding when you love what you do and pay that love forward."** Me too. I would like to raise a glass of Tuscan Chianti or Larry's coffee to all the women who have found, or are seeking, that special space. I wish us all a life of radiance and passion and joy.

12

Roots and Wings: Cherish the Past but Keep Growing

> "Don't cry because it's over. Smile because it happened."
>
> — Dr. Seuss

I TRULY LOVE this quote. Dr. Suess is a great favorite of mine and this is so like what I think of him: simple and winsome—and true. My children learned to value and play with words through *Cat in the Hat*, they were exposed to environmental responsibility through *The Lorax*, and they experienced compassion through *Horton Hatches the Egg*. This quote teaches me the wisdom of perspective and acceptance. These particular words of his also remind me of a song I love that has been extremely cathartic to me this year. I put on my CD of Garth Brooks singing "The Dance" and with tears in my eyes I sing along at the top of my lungs with the words, "I could have missed the pain, but I would have had to miss the dance." (I have to say it's even better if I'm simultaneously painting.) Just like Anais Nin's tightly closed little bud, if we aren't willing to open up to the storms and searing heat, we will never know the wonder of a soft spring breeze on our face.

This particular quote has meaning for me on a number of different levels and connects with many of the themes I have been writing about this year. So much of what was familiar in my life is over and I'm in a period of waiting for the next stage of my life to unfold. I become impatient and sometimes I am tortured with the fear that maybe I will <u>never</u> discover my next steps. Maybe I'll be circling the airport forever. But when I'm not feeling that frantic push to grab control and make something happen, I understand that this quiescent period is incredibly important. I am at least beginning to understand things about myself that have too long been beneath the surface. I am focusing on bringing more wholeness into my life. I am starting to come to terms with my flaws as well as celebrating my strengths. I have learned that I will never become the positive, joyful, fun-to-be-with woman I want to be as I grow older as long as I am bitter about what I no longer have. My physical and emotional well-being depend on not getting stuck in mourning what no longer is and opening my mind and my heart to what can be. Dr. Seuss' quote says all those things to me.

Much of my thinking has changed and evolved throughout this year, but there is still an elephant in the room. The reason it's the elephant in the room is that, as hard as it is to ignore it, it's even harder to talk about it, so I just step quietly around it feeling myself tense up if I get too close. That elephant for me is how to define my relationship with the school I retired from leading. I'm not sure I am alone in that dilemma. I think many of us worry about the protocol of retiring. Is the farewell party the end and then the door is closed on that place and the people who were once such a large part of your life? Do we ride off into the sunset or do we try to maintain some contact and, if so, what would that contact look like? As with all of this, there is no template we can follow. One of my husband's close friends retired as the Senior Minister of the major Presbyterian church in our city. Presbyterians have a rule that former ministers can have nothing to do with their former church for 3 years. They can't even enter the building. So that answers that question and there is no ambivalence. At the other end of the spectrum, I know a business owner who announced his retirement, named his successor and then proceeded to come to work every day as though nothing had changed. Most of us don't have guidelines, so we must work it out on our own.

    This has been a hugely problematic issue for me. When I am in Indianapolis I go back and forth in my mind as to whether I should stop by and visit the students and staff I knew so well. When I am aware of a major event I obsessively question whether I should attend. I want to stay out of the way and let the new leader lead and I also think it would make me sad to be there in such a different capacity. I do maintain contact with some of the parents who were also close friends and it is fun to have lunch with them and catch up on all that is going on. But when on occasion I see a former student they invariably say they miss me and wonder why I haven't come to visit them. I feel a certain amount of guilt when I don't visit because I wouldn't want to give the impression that I no longer care about the families and students I shared such a close bond with. It has been a year-long dilemma for me and I can't count the number of times I have made plans to stop by the school and then just simply couldn't do it at the last minute. I attended the dedication of the new building in October and have not been back since. The bottom line is that I'm not sure a visit from me would be welcomed by the new Head and his staff. And rightly so. It is their school to run now and it might be somewhat disconcerting to have the former Head—not to mention one who had frequently been referred to as "the face of the school"—wandering the halls.

    Back and forth—not wanting to interfere, but also not wanting to appear uncaring. I recognize that a large part of the problem is fueled by two ugly heads that rear up way too often in our lives and in these pages—worrying about what other people think and a fear of rejection. So words that may sound noble: "I want to stay out of the way of the new Head's efforts to establish his headship" can really mean: "What if I show up and it is embarrassing and awkward?" And then there is the lesson I learned on the ramparts. I really do miss the children, so am I allowing my fears to once again shut me out from something I really want to do? Am I singularly over-concerned about this? My guess is that unless you are a former Presbyterian minister or someone whose way is clearly laid out in your organization's policy manual, you may be also struggling to figure out what to do.

Then this whole angst-filled matter came to a head for me. I received an invitation to this year's graduation ceremony from a dear friend whose son is one of Midwest Academy's graduates. We have maintained contact over this year and she really wanted me to attend the ceremony because she was so proud of how far her son had come and she was grateful for the part I had played in his life. Because of that relationship I had no choice. I had to face the elephant.

I am so glad I went. My fears were unfounded. It was a very different ceremony from the ones I had conducted for seven years. It was held at a different location. Instead of the more formal and "fancy" venue we had always used, it was at the school. The format was extremely different, and there were not the same emotional vibes. The new Head is, wisely, creating his own traditions in a style that is far different from mine. These differences made the experience enough unlike the tradition that I knew that the occasion for me was not steeped in nostalgia and memories.

The graduates were happy I was there for their big moment and several underclassmen asked if I would please also come to their future graduations. I reconnected with parents I had not seen for awhile. In the midst of the hugs and the heartfelt statements that "we miss you" I felt closure. The experience was warm and comfortable. My presence did not create a distraction or drama. It was as though it was perfectly natural that I be there. I was embraced by the community and I felt reconnected although in a very different way. This experience did not make me feel that I need to do this more often. In fact, I felt more free to let it go. But it did serve as a powerful reminder of the good that I did and the lives that I changed and it brought back how much I have cared about these special students and their parents. I smiled when one of my former students, an extremely articulate 8th grader, said in his formal and ultra-serious way, "Dr Stoughton, we all miss you. We were used to seeing you in that office." I got a little misty-eyed when a sweet, almost silent boy who, at times, would speak only to me stood patiently in front of me with his loving and loyal grandmother waiting for me to notice him and congratulate him on graduating from 8th grade. I loved it when a bubbly middle school girl (who sang the entire aria from Phantom of the Opera complete with mask and cape at last year's talent show) threw her arms around me and announced, "I'm still singing. I knew you'd want to know that." Each of these children entered my life for awhile and I will never forget them. But there were many new faces there, children and families I didn't recognize and whose lives I had not been part of. And that will be increasingly true each year until there will no longer be anyone I knew. And that's all right. It's nothing more than the rhythm of life. I am starting to realize that there are moments in time, special seasons, when we make a difference in ways that only we can. But those powerful times don't have to continue on an on to be meaningful and to have worth. The ripples of them continue in ways that we aren't even aware of. I am proud of what I accomplished at that school and I hold many cherished memories in my heart. Right now as I'm writing this I am smiling because that time in my life happened and I am so tremendously grateful that I didn't miss that particular, very beautiful, dance.

13

The Only Good Place to Live is Outside the Box

"Creativity comes from looking for the unexpected and stepping outside your own experience."

— MASARU IBUKA

THE REALIZATION THAT I am almost at the end of my year's commitment of chronicling my journey into retirement makes me feel unsettled and a little nervous. This year has gone by so quickly and I still don't have complete clarity about where I stand or exactly where I am heading. I do know that through this process I have developed a level of self-awareness that I didn't have before. I can't say I have achieved wholeness in that regard. I think that's probably a lifetime job. But I do feel I am much more in touch with myself. I can even laugh at my flaws and failings on occasion, something I haven't always found easy to do. I am, however, a little cloudier about what other lasting learning and growth this year has brought me. I can say that I have been through many and varied experiences from a serious fall to being stuck in a snowdrift, but how exactly the year's experiences changed my life is still a bit vague.

I don't want to get ahead of myself as I plan to spend next month reflecting on recapping the year. But there is one theme that is unavoidable because it stands out so clearly. It is also a theme I think a lot about as I move into this last month of journaling. What I am talking about is the matter of creativity. I am thinking not only in terms of my discovery of pastel painting or as an encouragement to anyone who reads this to develop their "own inner Rembrandt (or Mozart, or Hemingway.)" I am looking at creativity in a much broader sense. I read Picasso's words, **"Every child is an artist. The problem is how to remain an artist once he grows up"** and I think those words refer to more than putting paint on canvas. I think they have to do with how we look at ourselves and our possibilities and potential. I believe they have to do with the number of amazingly talented adults who say "I'm not creative" and therefore shut themselves off from whole avenues of self-discovery. In fact, I'm coming to believe that our relationship to creativity and whether we believe we "have it" or not colors our worldview.

I am absolutely fascinated by innovative ideas and bold, imaginative thinkers. I can spend hours happily reading about unique discoveries and novel ways to solve problems. I love magazines like *Fast Company* because I am interested in their vignettes of people who have come up with ground-breaking ideas. My reaction generally falls into one of two categories, either "Why didn't I think of that?" or "Who could ever think of something like that?" depending on my level of experience with the subject. The mindset of so many of the featured people has an element of flexibility and vision that I think we all could benefit from. So I was thrilled to come across *Fast Company's* most recent edition featuring the "100 Most Creative People of the Year." What could possibly be better than spending a few hours finding out about innovators like the young woman who is doing her part to help get illegal guns off the streets by melting them down into trendy jewelry and contributing part of the proceeds to organizations working on street violence or the medical researcher who has developed an affordable, easy test for ovarian cancer that is dramatically increasing detection rates in Third World countries. This started me thinking about creativity in general. Is creativity a special quality reserved for impressionist painters and brilliant entrepreneurs? On the contrary, I am starting to believe that imaginative thinking **must** play a crucial role for each of us in our retirement lives. It makes so much sense to me. Much of this conversation has been about finding an alternative path between the career life we are no longer living and the traditional idea of retirement. Part of our struggle is against stereotypical and outdated notions of "our place" in society and what we can, and cannot, do. I like to think of us in this generation as "lifestyle change agents." The only answer, I believe, is to develop an innovative new path, one that fits who we are. To truly be trailblazers and venture into uncharted territory requires coming up with a creative vision. Psychologist Marie Forgeard of the University of Pennsylvania writes intriguingly in the journal *Scientific American Mind* (March/April 2014) that "**going through adversity may enable individuals to see the world, and their role in it, in a different way.**" She says that creative growth is stimulated by changes in our lives and that stressful circumstances have been shown to stimulate cognitive flexibility and open us up to being more creative. That is fascinating to me because it helps explain my sudden discovery of a heretofore hidden artistic side after all these years.

I am certainly not suggesting that in order to live a happy life any of us needs to do anything on the scope of melting guns into jewelry or inventing a process to combat cancer. So what creative thinking processes am I suggesting? I have compiled my top list of qualities that describe for me the core of creative living. From that list creativity is:

> Turning challenges into opportunities
> Doing things that I haven't done before
> Asking different questions
> Trusting my instincts
> Rethinking constraints
> Changing the lens

To sum up, according to a dear friend and partner in this journey, we need to:

> Retool
> Redefine
> Reinvent
> Re-Imagine

There has certainly been a major change in my life. The difference in the quality and direction of that change will clearly depend on whether I can do things that I have not done before. Changing my customary lens will help me discern the new path. I also know how important it is to re-imagine myself. Changing the self-pictures I carry in my head is crucial to changing my life. If I see myself as sitting on the sidelines, that is where I will be. Far better I think to, as a young woman CEO said, **"stay agile and adapt."** Although my agility may be a bit questionable on some days, I do think that adapting is extraordinarily important.

A recent advertisement aired on television asks the question, **"Shouldn't retirement be about doing what we love?"** Absolutely. It seems to me that a good life would consist of settling on what we love doing and finding a way to do it that works with who we are and what we are able to do. Sometimes the way is already paved for us to be able to do what we love doing because there is a structure already created to fit into. For example, a member of the group that came together to discuss these issues has been a highly esteemed and beloved teacher at the same school for over 30 years. She retired this spring and is inundated with requests to continue working with students by tutoring them. She greatly enjoys tutoring, so this is a natural for her. In other cases it isn't so simple. If structures aren't already in place, we need to get to work to first define our purpose and then look at ways we can carry that purpose out. Sometimes that will require forging a new pathway, one that hasn't been thought of before. It will definitely take self-awareness and a mind open to previously unthought-of possibilities.

Although the first step—defining your purpose—sounds like the easy part, it can be surprisingly difficult to center on what you truly want to do. Many of us have not received a lot of encouragement in our lives to put our wants and needs first. There isn't always a priority placed on being reflective about what you would like to do. I do think, however, that there is something for everyone although sometimes it may be buried deeply in the wistful part of our being where sentences start out "If only..." I also don't think it has to be just one thing. One of the beauties of retirement is that we are able to explore and enjoy a variety of experiences. In fact, some research studies show that women tend to be healthiest and happiest when we take on a variety of roles. The things I love are making art, working with other women to live our best lives forward (and, of course finishing this book) and supporting children with disabilities and their families. I want to continue to pursue all of them. My problem lies more in the next step—coming up with a creative plan for each of these. Or, maybe it would be better to say that I haven't yet come up with a plan that has reached completion and that works well. As the saying goes, **a goal is a dream with a timeline.** I have always been far more proficient with the dreaming than with the timeline. But I'm becoming more focused on how to make what I care about happen. It hasn't been easy. I become discouraged and disheartened and lose my enthusiasm for forging ahead with new ideas. "It won't work" pops too easily out of my mouth. I am my own worst critic, and perfectionism dogs my steps. But on the other hand, I believe in the rightness and truth of my dreams and am confident in myself and my ability to make those dreams come true. One thing I've learned this year for sure is that living a life without purpose or focus and having too much time on my hands is not healthy for me or, for that matter, anyone who has to put up with me. I embody the person Howard Schultz, Starbucks CEO, was thinking of when he said, **"If you don't**

have passion, you don't have any energy. If you don't have energy you don't have anything." It makes sense to me that, as a number of research studies show, the narrowing of interests and resulting loss of enthusiasm and curiosity can be causes of dementia and depression.

One of my painting friends, Sue, embodies the power of passion and enthusiasm. A former university library science professor and author, Sue is now 91 years old. She lives in a charming log cabin on Lake Michigan where she cares lovingly for her husband who is slipping into a hazy state of loss of memory. She spends time with her many friends and she creates watercolor paintings. She is funny and blunt. One morning a small group of us were painting at the edge of a beautiful garden. One of the artists was trying to tell a story when Sue turned to her and said, "You know, I can't hear a darned thing a lot of the time, but I'll trust you that it's a funny story." She loves her art and her pride is apparent when she shows people proudly through her house where the walls are covered with her paintings. Sue could have plenty of reasons to feel sorry for herself. In the winter her little cabin can be pretty isolated, her beloved husband requires almost constant care, and—as she says—her hearing is not great. Yet, I have never heard a self-pitying word from her. She loves life and her spark is contagious.

As I mentioned earlier, I am becoming much more self-aware. I have come to know myself well enough to know that being inactive and uninvolved for too long spells trouble for me. So I have no choice. I have to commit to making my dreams come true for my own happiness and wellbeing. I have a feeling there are others of you who are reading this who also realize this about yourselves. I believe we are all meant to be involved and work hard and feel the wind beneath our wings when we create something we care about.

I am discovering that there is a delicate balance between quiet contemplation and focused action. That is why both finding what you love to do and then figuring out what to do to make it happen are equally important. We need to take time out to let the waves of imagination and contemplation wash over our minds in order to gain wisdom and discernment and a sense of what is true for us.

Most of us lean more in one direction than the other and that's the value of taking some time to work toward achieving that harmonious yin and yang in our lives. When I ask women to describe the biggest challenge for them in their retirement years, a surprisingly large number of them mentioned being too busy and scattered. As one woman put it, "I'm doing so many things and I'm not able to stop. I need to get off the gerbil wheel." Another woman added that she spends most of her time "doing and responding." A third response was simply that her problem was "too much busyness." Not that there is anything wrong with being busy. In fact some of my happiest and most fulfilled times were when I was totally absorbed in something I cared about and there never seemed to be quite enough time. However, my memories of times when I was feeling awash in busyness just to fill time or as a result of my own guilt and heavy sense of obligation are less happy. Guilt is a great motivator, it is just not a particularly positive one. I am not advocating a life of self-absorbed selfishness, but for most of us women there is little danger of that. What I am saying is that we need to balance our roles of nurturing and caretaking with honoring and respecting ourselves enough to live our lives on our own terms. What we give our time to should matter to us and we should be wholehearted about it.

My hope is that we all give ourselves permission to dream big and claim our inherent creativity to figure out a way to make those dreams come true. I hope that we can step out of our familiar experience; regard "conventional wisdom" with critical skepticism; give little credence to "the way it's always been done;" be willing to take risks; and wipe the phrase "I'm not creative" from our vocabulary.

Our dreams and what we can do with them are too important to lose.

It is so much easier to say "I am (a teacher, an attorney, a CEO) than it is to say, "I'm doing the hard inner work of trying to get in touch with who I really am so I can live a full and joyful life." And yet, I think that if, upon leaving full-time work, I had gotten my wish and jumped right into the same sort of life I have been used to and comfortable with, it would have been pretty much the same song, second verse and I would never do the inner work I needed to do to be truly contented. But it has not been a walk in the park. I met recently for coffee with one of my partners on this path who seems to always have a meaningful and encouraging word for me. Once again, she lazered in on just what I needed to hear when she said, "What you are doing now is lonely, solitary work. It's like gardening. You plant a garden and then you have to put in the hard work so it can grow, and you do it alone. But at the end the beauty of what you have created makes it all worthwhile. You are working on your own garden." The more I thought about those words, the more meaningful they were to me in giving me the belief that there is a purpose in all the weeding and cultivating I seem to keep doing. This must be a lesson I am supposed to learn because it was only a day later when I came across these words by Monroe Forester, **"Hope is always available to us. When we feel defeated, we need only take a deep breath and say, "yes" and hope will reappear."** Now I would be the first to admit that I am pretty far from Zen-like, but those words are incredibly meaningful to me and the more I turn them over in my mind the more meaning they have. In thinking about this, I am led to the question of what makes me feel defeated in the first place? It is probably different for each of us, but I believe that I experience those feelings when I feel I have missed the mark. I fear that I'm not doing what I should be doing and therefore, I'm not in the right place. Reminding myself of my long-term battle with perfectionism and my tendency to be hard on myself makes it pretty clear why I sometimes feel "down." But then the second question this quote leads me to ponder is, where does renewed hope come from? I have begun to realize that hope is born out of knowing that, whether I like it or not, I am in the place I should be for right now. I'm not in charge. I can drop the reins without fearing that everything will fall apart. As Anne Lamotte says, we need to stop grabbing on with our sticky, grasping fingers. I cannot express how amazing—and freeing—that realization is to me. It shakes the way I have always lived my life and makes me question the voice in my head that repeats, "You make your own fate, your future is in your hands and you have to take charge if you expect to make things happen. Therefore you have no one to blame but yourself if it goes badly." I do believe that retirement is a process not an event, but that only carries me so far. I think what I believed in was a time-limiting process that I would be able to zip through, learn some much-needed lessons to make my life smoother and then move on to the "important stuff" like embarking on my next big role. Yet, preparing the soil and pruning and weeding are absolutely necessary. I conveniently keep skipping over the cultivation part of my garden while I wait impatiently for the beautiful bouquet to arrive in my arms. It may just take a bit more time and I may need to learn more about saying "yes" to where I find myself.

14

A Year of Challenges, Growth, and Joy
One Year After the Date of My Retirement: July, 2014

"If you want to make God laugh, tell him your plans."

— Woody Allen

I HAVE COME to the end of the first year of my post-career life and I am a little sad because this anniversary marks the end of my commitment to write my monthly reflections. Getting my thoughts down on paper has been incredibly therapeutic and has led to rich and valuable connections with other women who are fellow travelers on this path. I will miss it.

My plan all along has been to sum up in this last entry the lessons I have learned and share a travelogue of the new ventures I have embarked on, forecasting where I am heading in the next years. But it is hard to know where to begin. True to my teacher self I would like to be able to present a meaningful lesson with universal applications and clear "takeaways." However, I don't feel I have achieved that sort of sure knowledge. The dots are still not all connected. The thing I do feel very sure about is that this is important work that we all inevitably must do, and that it takes time. I have discussed these issues with many women in widely different circumstances and all of them recognize the common experiences of complexity of emotions and perplexity about where to go from here. Although some of us have adapted to this new lifestyle more smoothly and easily while others of us are more angst-ridden, we all have in common a desire to live happy and meaningful lives and we want to be able to look forward to our future with optimism and enthusiasm. We just aren't always exactly sure what that means or how to make it happen.

As I look back over this past year, it hardly seems possible that one year ago I was giving my farewell speech at my final board meeting and posing for snapshots with board members. I was off to Michigan and the beginning of a very different life. I began filling suitcases and boxes for relocation with a mixture of feelings. On one hand, I felt unencumbered and free as this would be the first time I would be making this trip without also packing a full briefcase, a "to-do" list, and pages of email and phone contacts. On the other hand, I felt apprehensive about what shape my life would take. My uncertainty was fueled by the echoes of the words of an already retired well-wisher who jovially sent me off with the words, "You're going to love retirement. I don't do much of anything. In fact, the only way I can tell one day from the other is that Sunday has the fat paper." Although I knew that was not what I wanted, those who have been part of this journey from the beginning know it didn't take long before I hit the shoals coming uncomfortably close to a "fat paper Sunday" lifestyle. I became angry. The object of my anger was the aging process—its inevitably and unfairness. I wasn't ready. There was too much still to do. This getting older thing was an aberration and an indignity, a cruel trick that had been foisted upon me when I wasn't paying attention. But then I realized that being sad and mad was keeping me stuck. That was the beginning of my commitment to chronicle this unknown journey and, in so doing, hopefully get a handle on it.

In summing up, I have thought deeply about what I have learned this year. There are four major "takeaways" that I would like to share with you.

The first lesson begins with a story about sailing and the connection between steering a boat through the waves and leading a purposeful life.

Takeaway #1:

> "If a man knows not to which port he sails,
> no wind is favorable."
>
> — Seneca

This sailing metaphor speaks to me because I love sailing. I have always had a completely unrealistic, "bucket list" dream of crewing on one of the big racing sailboats. The closest I came was that for a number of years we had a little bright yellow Sunfish in Michigan that we affectionately called the Banana Boat. As much as I love sailing, however, I am a notoriously inept sailor. I have no real control of the process and so there have been times without number when the boat simply bobbed around aimlessly unable to head anywhere or became grounded unnervingly on the beach despite my most heroic efforts to turn it around. However, when I did manage to catch the wind, the feeling of skimming gracefully across the waves with the wind in my face was pure joy. It is a wonderful feeling. There is no better feeling than having somewhere we are heading and feeling that we are getting there with the wind at our backs. This thought is expressed by the words I recently read in our small town Michigan paper following the annual regatta:

> "Sailing a boat calls for quick action,
> a blending of feeling with the wind
> and water as well as with the very
> heart and soul of the boat itself.
> Sailing teaches alertness and courage,
> and gives in return a
> joyousness and peace that but few sports afford."
>
> — George Matthew Adams

That joy and optimism and sense of exhilaration is what I want for all of us. But this year with all its surprises, discoveries, doubts and fears has convinced me that sailing happily into the future isn't as effortless as it sounds.

One might ask why, in spite of my desires, I am such an unskilled sailor that I flounder trying to navigate a little one-sailed boat. The reason is that I bought the boat on an impulse and, having never had any instruction, I thought I would "pick it up as I went along." Sometimes it worked and other times not. Unfortunately, that is not far from the way I approached retirement, but the stakes were much higher. Oh, I had thought about it and believed I was formulating a plan, but it was a vague plan and I was pretty unrealistic about how it would all play out. I have come to the realization that I have lived my life pretty unconsciously, maintaining a pace that didn't allow for much introspection. So I embarked on this new phase of life with some unformed ideas of who I really am and what lifestyle would be the best fit for me. My romanticized picture of spending the year at our remote home in Michigan fully experiencing the change of seasons did not sufficiently include acknowledgement of how isolating it can be to be snowed in with no lights on in any houses for miles and with groceries and medical services over 30 miles away. I did love much of that experience as I wrote earlier, but that doesn't change the fact that I had no idea what I was getting into.

So, the first takeaway this year brought me is especially for those of you who are reading this before you retire. **Take plenty of reflective time to picture yourself in your planned future and note how it feels to you. Talk to people who have experienced it. Do your research. Be brutally honest with yourself. Don't be afraid to dig deeply to get to the core of your unique strengths and needs. Don't get caught up in an unrealistic, rosy-colored vision of how things will be.** If your experience is like mine, you will never achieve complete self-awareness, but the more mindful and intentional you are, the better the chances are that you will make wise choices. On the other hand, don't be afraid to dream boldly and get in touch with what will make you whole and complete. And take heart from women who have gone before us and have shown us what bold dreaming can mean. Each of those trailblazers has paved the way for us. A few examples include Grandma Moses who produced her first painting at the age of 76 and painted every day of her life until her death at 101, Laura Ingalls Wilder whose *Little House on the Prairie* series was written when in her 60s, Mother Teresa who was 69 years old when she won the Pulitzer Peace Prize and all the unheralded women who do courageous and amazing things on a regular basis.

Of course, as I have written, the experience of retirement itself has made looking deeply within myself unavoidable and there are lessons I could not have learned ahead of time no matter how meticulously and wisely I planned. But how much better to head into the wind from the beginning of the voyage and then make course corrections as necessary along the way. The time to begin to re-imagine yourself is now.

Takeaway #2:

> "Every blade of grass has its angel bending over it whispering, "Grow, grow!"
>
> — THE TALMUD

The connection between art and life forms the backdrop for my second lesson.

Last week I signed up for a two-day plein air painting workshop that was taught by an accomplished artist who lives near our home in Michigan. To those who are not familiar with the term, plein air painting simply means landscape painting that is done on-site and outdoors rather than in a studio. I was looking forward greatly to the experience, not only because I knew I would learn much about painting, but also because the teacher is a friend of mine. It was a truly pleasurable and enlightening two days and, as I anticipated, I learned invaluable skills thanks to the wise coaching of the teacher, Heidi.

The first day of the workshop was a beautiful sunny day and we set up our easels in a park-like setting on the shore of Lake Michigan. I couldn't wait to dive in. I picked my spot and was working industriously when I realized that Heidi was standing behind me looking over my shoulder. She began to gently critique what I was doing. My first thought was to be a little hurt—I have mentioned how important affirmation is to me—but then I started to listen with an open mind to what she was telling me. She asked me to put down my pastels and just sit and feel with my senses. Very simply what Heidi was telling me was to be aware and to be in the moment. I sat for quite a while (it felt like an eternity) with the summer breeze on my face and I began to notice details of the scene that I had been too busy diving in to notice before. It looked very different from my first impression—fuller, richer, more vibrant. There was a soft shade of violet in the shadows that I had missed and the clouds were far more beautiful and interesting than I had realized. The longer I sat and just let my surroundings sink into my consciousness the more I began to feel at one with the scene. It was exhilarating. I was really "there" instead of on the periphery observing and dashing to get it on paper.

The next day we painted on the edge of farm fields. My approach this time was very different. I sat for a long time just absorbing what was around me. It was hard not to start splashing color on paper. It required a self-discipline I don't always possess. But I did it and as time ticked by I was captured by the complete silence and peace. I heard an insect buzzing nearby and I was surprised by the many different colors of green there are in trees. But I was also learning about myself and how nice it is to slow down. This time when I started painting I wasn't thinking of creating an impressive finished product. I was absorbed in the simple joy of representing what I saw and felt.

So this is the second life lesson I am learning—to be able to sit and wait and absorb what is around me. To take the time I need to be patient with myself and the process and not expect to have everything figured out and all the ends tied up on my timetable. I need to learn to be comfortable with uncertainty and to value the questions that present themselves rather than jumping to the answers—<u>any</u> answers to remove the discomfort of feeling adrift. I am learning so much about myself during this process and some of the things I am learning are uncomfortable. But it is necessary that I understand them if I am going to grow.

One of the more uncomfortable things I am learning involves negative self-talk. Most of us have a word (or more) that can be incredibly wounding when we use it against ourselves. For some women that word is "fat." Calling themselves fat is a self-flagellating experience of disapproval and shame. For other women it may be "ugly" or "stupid." For many of us, ironically, that word is "old." Sadly, there are any number of these types of negative words that stem from the **shame turned inward** that Brene Brown speaks and writes about. For me, the word is "lazy." I am not quite sure why the idea of laziness holds such negative connotations for me. It most probably has to do with my hard-working, no-nonsense forbears: farmers, small town bankers, business owners who lived by the adage that "idle hands are the devil's workshop." Whatever the reason, this word holds such sway over me, if I believe that I am being lazy I have intense feelings of guilt and worthlessness and it frightens me. That has made the process of slowing down and getting in touch with myself particularly hard because I can't always emotionally distinguish between being content in saying "yes" to my present circumstances and being "just plain lazy." If I believe that the opposite of being driven is being lazy then I desperately search for a way to become driven again because a high level of stress is certainly preferable to being lazy. So being able to value calm and quiet reflection and feeling comfortable with where I am without the need to be constantly doing something is also an important part of what I needed to learn. I am getting better. I can now actually enjoy a lovely day guilt free with no specific goal other than enjoying it. I have also made a promise that I will stop punishing myself with words. I would invite any of you who have a similar problem to join with me in that promise.

I believe that the key message that the angel who is bending over me is whispering in my ear is, "Growing for you means giving up concerns about your reputation and what people think of you and becoming comfortable in your own skin." Many of my accomplishments and goals throughout my life have been formulated with other people's reactions in mind. Making a big impression has always been important to me. So the best retirement gift I can give myself is to free myself from the heavy expectations that have seemed to be an unavoidable part of my life for so long and to give myself permission to set my own path. **I believe that the most valuable thing about retirement is that we are given the opportunity to step back and define OUR OWN goals, OUR OWN priorities and OUR OWN vision.** We are not disappearing or retreating from life, we are taking a temporary hiatus to reinvent, retool and redefine ourselves. We have a special opportunity to connect with what we really care about and what matters to us. The very thing that makes us uncomfortable about being retired—our lack of involvement in the matters that used to consume us—is what give us that opportunity to do the inner work that can lead to self-knowledge. We have been given the gift of time as well as a lifetime of wisdom and experience to help us use that time wisely. What seems at the moment to be the curse of a life sentence to oblivion is really a blessing. But in order to reap that blessing, we will have to value **being** over **doing.** We will have to be open and eager to learn even if the learning is painful and hard. But it is worth it because self-knowledge and self-respect are the tools we need to begin living our best lives forward. And that takes time and patience.

My first takeaway was about the importance of readying ourselves as much as possible for this transition through honest and mindful reflection and planning. The second concerned taking time to know our authentic selves by having patience with the process and learning what we need to learn. It is about giving ourselves the space to listen and think and to be gentle with ourselves on this voyage of discovery. If we do that, we will be healthier, happier and more whole. This brings me to the third lesson I would like to share. It may be the most important because it has to do with the outcome of that preparation and mindfulness. It is about who we want to become and what we want to accomplish in the coming years.

Takeaway #3:

> "If the world puts you on a road you do not like, if you look ahead and do not want that destination that is being offered, and you look behind and you do not want to return to your place of departure, step off the road. Build yourself a brand new path."
>
> — MAYA ANGELOU ATTRIBUTED THESE WORDS TO HER GRANDMOTHER

Maya Angelou was someone whose dignity, wisdom and grace defined for me, and for countless others, what growing older gracefully means. She was a force for truth until her death and her influence will continue long into the future. When I read her grandmother's words of strength, purpose and resolve, I understand the foundation for her character.

This powerful quotation should be emblazoned on our hearts and inscribed on a plaque to hang in our homes because it expresses exactly what so many of us think and feel at this time in our lives. Although there are things we might miss about our former life, most of us don't really want to go back there. Many of us don't like the destination that is being offered to us: retirement living as traditionally understood, fat Sunday paper and all. So we have no other choice but to build a new path.

Earlier I shared my friend's advice about the important work of preparing a garden. The part about being willing to do the solitary work needed to produce the beautiful result was necessary for me to hear. However, my friend would say that, as important as the preparation is, the whole point is to end up with a garden. One doesn't prepare endlessly with no result in mind and nothing to show for all that work and effort.

A related analogy would be creating pottery. My oldest daughter, Amanda, and I enrolled in a pottery class together at our local art league one summer. It soon became clear that Amanda had real natural ability in this area and I didn't. (Although there are a number of things I can do well, sailing and pottery are not two of them.) The whole key is in getting the wet clay centered on the wheel in the beginning. Centering provides the foundation and strength that supports the rest of the creation. Bending over wet clay to carefully mold it with your hands is a lengthy and difficult process particularly when you are anxious to get on to the "fun part." But the most beautiful pot will topple over if not centered properly on the wheel. I could never seem to get the feel of it no matter how hard I tried. Amanda was a natural. Her pots stood straight and tall and beautiful while my wobbly creations simply crumpled in upon themselves. And yet, analogous to the garden, as crucial and necessary as the centering is, the whole point of the process is to produce a finished piece of pottery.

Neither of these processes can be rushed, but there is a reason for all that patient, careful work. First, we step off the road and open our hearts to learn about ourselves and our purpose and then we build our own unique path. Without building the path, we would be simply standing endlessly by the side of the road with no destination in mind and nowhere to go.

I have kept personal journals for years. One of my most cherished extravagances is to periodically treat myself to a lovely new leather journal and record my thoughts in it. I have journals devoted entirely to quotes that are meaningful to me and other journals cataloguing difficult or joyful times in my life. It is eye opening to look back through my journals and read what I was thinking years ago. As I was reading back through my 2010-2011 journal I came upon a page with a statement I had written that simply said, **"I REFUSE TO LET ANYONE DEFINE ME"** in giant letters that filled the page.

I still believe that and I would still use giant letters. I would now, four years later, add that if I don't want anyone else to define me, then I must define myself on my own terms and in my own way.

That's really the point I keep coming back to. I think that we all have a deep desire for something that defines us. I truly believe that each of us is meant to find something we love to do and do it with our whole heart. I also trust that we will know what that is because we will have a conviction that comes from the time we have spent centering. Writing this has helped me open my eyes to what I need to see about myself and my place in the world. I still don't understand everything, but I feel that each day I am closer to being ready to walk through new doors and make new memories. That brings me back to the need to look at things creatively. **Building a new path takes boldness and imagination. It means saying "yes" to the voice that comes from inside you and "no" to the mold that the world would like to put you in. It means taking risks and being willing to fail. It**

means not being devastated if you look foolish and being the first one to laugh at your foibles and mistakes. Mostly it means being kind and gentle with yourself and trusting your inner wisdom.

I came across something else I had written when I was reading through some of my old journals. On June 3, 2012 I wrote, "I want to do something that is lasting and beautiful." I still do. I don't know yet what it will be, but I am excited to watch it unfold.

Takeaway #4:

> "Alone we can do so little, together we can do so much."
>
> — Helen Keller

The fourth, and final, area I would like to talk about concerns our relationship with each other. I admit I was a bit surprised to discover that Helen Keller wrote those words as my picture of her has always tended to be that of a strong individualist who made her way in a hearing and seeing world through sheer grit and determination. But clearly she saw things differently and through my own journey I am beginning to understand why.

Whoever said that growing old is not for sissies was telling the truth. We need each other for strength, inspiration and companionship. Sheryl Sandberg and the work she is doing with **Lean In** has shown us that having supporters, encouragers and exemplars can make an incredible difference in the lives of working women. If these assertive, on-the-way-up career women benefit from that support, so can we. We learn from, and draw strength from, each other. In addition to the companionship that quite a few of us already have developed in social and friendship groups, I believe there is an additional need for something more purposeful. We need support groups of women who have a commitment to care enough to encourage us and hold us to account. We need our own form of **Lean In** to push us forward. Who better to do that than other women who understand our situation on a personal basis.

Retirement can be lonely and we can miss the way a set schedule once organized our days. I remember clearly the day I woke up in the morning and realized there was nowhere I had to be—and not just for that day, but from then on. First I felt the same excitement I felt as a child—and as a teacher—when I was given the gift of a snow day with school cancelled and nothing I had to do but enjoy it. Then I felt unmoored. In a throwback to the stock phrase, "I do it myself" that I repeated constantly at two-years old, and that in those days led to clothes on backwards and shoes placed on the wrong feet, I started out with a grim determination to meet the challenges and to make a success of this part of my life on my own. I was determined to prove I could meet the challenges by myself. Anything less was a form of weakness. Then I realized—with relief—that there is strength in togetherness and that most things are better when they are shared with others who are dealing with the same issues. This is not an experience that goes better if one is lonely, isolated and disconnected.

During my lifetime I have seen countless examples of women who wanted something different for their lives and came together to change society's expectations. I can proudly say that I was part of some of those changes. Our generation successfully challenged the common thinking that women could aspire to be nurses but not doctors, secretaries but not CEOs and teachers but not Heads of School. We altered the dominant opinion that a woman's role is to support her husband and that it is unseemly to have her own ambitions. We demonstrated that women can have fulfilling work lives outside the home without abandoning their children or destroying their family life. I believe that together we can clear the next hurdle: to change society's ideas of what retired women can be and what we can accomplish. Contrary to the popular opinion that we have "retired" in its classical meaning of quietly going away, we have so much to offer that is lying dormant and just needs encouragement to blossom. Many of us are already blooming! I know a number of women who are doing extraordinary things. One woman I know says simply that she loves projects. A retired executive with strong organizational abilities, she throws herself into a wide range of projects that bring amazing benefit to causes she cares about. A retired teacher of my acquaintance is writing the children's book she has wanted to write for years. Another woman teaches yoga to children with disabilities, basing her work on research that shows the positive affects of yoga training on the concentration and wellbeing of children with learning and neurological differences. Running for office, starting a small business that trains and hires previously unemployed workers and driving a food truck in a remote rural area to bring healthy meals to families living in poverty are all ways the retired women I know are making a difference. We can contribute by giving them our encouragement and support. **We need to be each others' cheerleaders and coaches. So let us take Helen Keller's words to heart and never overlook the need to join together to lift each other up. We are not finished, we are just beginning. Together we are a force!**

I would like to revisit the story I told in the beginning about my friend who had to leave her career due to health problems and the group she became part of. Recently, while looking back through my old journals I came across the journal entry I wrote on the day she told me the story in 2011. I think it's important to hear it in her own words.

My Journal Entry. June 7, 2011:
She admitted that she floundered for a while after she became ill, not knowing what to do and feeling lost. Then one day she ran into a woman she knew, but not well. This woman had been diagnosed with breast cancer and she too had to leave her high-profile job. And that was when the agreement was made to start meeting every two weeks to get away for a brief time from what they were dealing with

and to enjoy a fun activity together. They said they would do this until they found something that gave purpose to their lives, something that would take precedence. Other women heard about them and joined them. The group became 6. They met faithfully for several years and then gradually, one-by-one, they started dropping out. But it wasn't a bad thing—it was as it should be and as was planned in the beginning. Each one found the purpose she had been looking for. Finally it returned to the original two. My friend helped the other woman fulfill her dream of starting a little knit shop. But what was my friend's goal? She told me her goal is simply to do the good she can knowing that she makes a difference that way. She emphasized that she doesn't miss the title or accolades, that just knowing within herself what she is doing is what matters. Her final words were: Women **always** find a way to connect.

Final Thought:

> Wheresoever you go, go with all your heart.
>
> — CONFUCIUS

This month I had my own booth at a local art fair near our home in Michigan. I filled out the application, bought a canopy, and stocked my booth with boxes of note cards I had made from my paintings. I purposefully chose paintings of local sites that people living there would recognize, and hopefully, identify with, to make my cards more sellable. I had no inkling of how much I would enjoy the experience. My choice of local landmarks proved to be a good one as many people stopped by my booth to talk about the places I had chosen. They reminisced about their connection with the sites and told fascinating stories. One young couple said they had been married on a beach scene I had chosen and they just wanted to buy that one particular card rather than a whole box as a memory of that joyful event. All in all it was an extremely enjoyable day. I sold more than I thought I would and met many friendly people in the process.

The very best part of the day was that I had the opportunity to share the booth with my 9-year old granddaughter, Ana. Ana had crafted notebooks with specially designed pockets to hold pens attached to the front. They were very clever and useful and she and her mother had spent a great deal of time picking out the fabric and trim and putting the pockets on the notebooks. I told her she could have half of my table to display her products and she was thrilled to be able to participate. She planned on giving 10% of her earnings to an autism association in honor of her brother, Nate. People loved her notebooks and her goal to help autism on behalf of her brother. But most of all they loved her enthusiasm and heart. The fair opened at 10 AM and she had sold all of her notebooks by noon! She was elated and full of excitement at the amazing day she had been part of and we are already making plans for next year's event.

A year ago I would not have pictured myself selling note cards from my own booth space at an art fair. It would have seemed quite out of character. But that was before I experienced this year with all its ups-and-downs and surprising lessons. I have learned so much about thinking differently about things and making peace with who I am and where I am in my growth and learning. I am increasingly able to be in the moment and savor the simple joy of sharing an experience like this with my beloved granddaughter. I can give myself permission to completely throw myself into the moment without any thought that I should be doing something more meaningful and earth-changing than participating in a local art fair. Additionally, I have joined a group of several ladies who paint together every Tuesday morning and I am now able to walk the beach without a pen and paper in my hand to make sure I record any profound thoughts or to-do items that might happen to occur to me at the water's edge. I am discovering that life is good and that my life has profound meaning. I feel relaxed, happy and peaceful a much greater amount of time than I have before. I would still love to "hit one out of the ball park." I still have a deep desire to make a difference. But I am emotionally prepared now to stand back and watch what develops, trusting in the process rather than feeling the urgency to jump into anything that sounds good and has the opportunity to return me once again to prominence. It feels like the difference between running **from** and running **toward.** Before, I was anxiously running from the fear of becoming insignificant and invisible. Now I am moving toward my own personally meaningful definition of significance. I am increasingly aware of the importance of balance. Plans collapse like my crumpled ceramic pots if we aren't first centered, but we need equally much the vitality and enthusiasm that come from commitment and challenge. Although the world would like to convince us otherwise, it is never too late to dream or to plan for our next steps. I am challenged by a question I read not too long ago: **"What gets you up in the morning and what keeps you up at night?"** We each have to answer that question in our own way, but the answer can make a difference in our lives.

I don't mean to give the false impression that I have gained so much equilibrium and insight this year that my life has become a Hallmark card. There is still work to do. There are days when I worry that I'm becoming complacent and that I'm "settling." I am still on the search for meaning and significance and the fact that I have the most "stubbornly arrhythmic heart" my cardiologist says he has ever seen makes the concept of blooming where I am planted somewhat more challenging. But I sat recently on our deck basking in the quiet and beauty of a blazing sunset. I was surrounded by silence that was only broken by the distant eerie call of a loon. As the sun dipped below the surface of Lake Michigan I took a few minutes to think about some of the things I now know that I didn't always consciously know before. I now know in my heart that with the love and respect of my husband, my children and my grandchildren, I will never become invisible. After spending vacation time in Michigan with my granddaughters Campbell and Lauren, Campbell said to her mother that "Nana is the best teacher." I can believe in my heart that this is as worthwhile as teaching a whole class (or school) of students. I know that I can be happy and just simply enjoy my days without feeling guilty that I'm not doing something judged important in the eyes of the world. I know that gathering with friends to take this journey together and possibly even be someone who helps point the way is both important and rewarding work. I know that being happy doing things you love to do with people you love to be with is a worthwhile occupation. Most of all, I know that I will never willingly let anyone define me and that my value comes from inside me. I still have enticing ideas of things I would like to do percolating in my head. I love thinking about them. Some are good ideas, but not right for me at this time, others are intriguing and deserve exploration. I still feel that I am on the cusp of something. I love the idea of writing about my journey further and so I hope to write periodic follow-ups. That is something to look forward to.

I wish for each of you that you find your own way to happiness and significance. As my friend said, just personally knowing that what she was doing made a difference was enough for her. We are all important and have valuable contributions that no one else can make. And we can still have so much to do and to become if we always believe in ourselves. I believe that one of the most destructive phrases we can utter is, "It's too late for me." It is never too late!

To sum up, I would like to share with you the familiar and yet always beautiful and touching words that a little boy once said to his best friend, a bumbly little stuffed bear:

> Promise me you'll always remember: You're braver than you believe, stronger than you seem, and smarter than you think."
>
> — Christopher Robin to Winnie the Pooh

About the Author

Dr. Edy Stoughton has been a special education teacher, administrator, and head of school in both private and public schools for over 30 years. After earning her doctorate at Indiana University, Bloomington in 2001, she taught at the University level at Teacher's College, Columbia University and Indiana University, Indianapolis and served as Head of School for Midwest Academy in Carmel, Indiana. She is the mother of 5 children and the grandmother of 5 grandchildren. Dr. Stoughton retired in 2014 and now she spends most of her time in Northern Michigan with her husband Steve and their Goldendoodle, Chance where she writes and creates art.

She has had a number of articles published in educational and sociology journals, but this is her first book.

Made in the USA
Las Vegas, NV
17 July 2023